The Cultures of Caregiving

Thomas H. Murray, consulting editor in bioethics

The Cultures of Caregiving

Conflict and Common Ground among
Families, Health Professionals, and
Policy Makers

Edited by

Carol Levine, M.A.
Director, Families and Health Care Project
United Hospital Fund
New York, New York

and

Thomas H. Murray, Ph.D.
President, The Hastings Center
Garrison, New York

Foreword by Christine K. Cassell, M.D.

The Johns Hopkins University Press
Baltimore and London

The Johns Hopkins University Press
2715 North Charles Street
Baltimore, Maryland 21218-4363
www.press.jhu.edu

Library of Congress Cataloging-in-Publication Data

The cultures of caregiving: conflict and common ground among families,
health professionals, and policy makers / edited by Carol Levine and
Thomas H. Murray ; with a foreword by Christine K. Cassel.
   p. ; cm.
Includes bibliographical references and index.
   ISBN 0-8018-7863-2 (hardcover : alk. paper)
   1. Home care services.   2. Chronically ill—Home care.   3. Aged—Home
care.   4. Caregivers—Psychology.   5. Home nursing—Psychological
aspects.   6. Family nursing.   7. Nurse and patient.
   [DNLM: 1. Caregivers—psychology.   2. Home Nursing—psychology.
3. Family Relations.   4. Professional-Family Relations.   WY 200 C967 2004]
I. Levine, Carol. II. Murray, Thomas H., 1946–
   RA645.3.C85 2004
   362.14—dc22

                                                          2003016414

A catalog record for this book is available from the British Library.

Contents

Contributors

Donna Jean Appell, R.N., is a cofounder and codirector of Project DOCC: Delivery of Chronic Care. She is also the founder and president of the Hermansky-Pudlak Syndrome Network, Inc. (Hermansky-Pudlak syndrome is a genetic disorder that is characterized by albinism, low vision, and a bleeding problem. Some genetic mutations can cause inflammatory bowel disease and pulmonary fibrosis.) She is a member of the board of directors of the Genetic Alliance, the educational coordinator for Reach Out for Youth with Ileitis and Colitis, and a board member and medical advisory board member for the National Organization for Albinism and Hypopigmentation. Donna Appell has worked as an open-heart cardiac intensive care unit nurse at St. Francis Hospital, Roslyn, New York, since 1982. She has two children, one of whom is living with Hermansky-Pudlak syndrome.

Jeffrey Blustein, Ph.D., is a professor of bioethics at the Albert Einstein College of Medicine and a clinical bioethicist at Montefiore Medical Center, Bronx, New York. He also teaches ethics and medicine at Barnard College, where he is an adjunct associate professor. Blustein is the author of two books on ethics, *Parents and Children: The Ethics of the Family* (1982) and *Care and Commitment: Taking the Personal Point of View* (1991). He is coauthor, with Nancy Dubler and Linda Farber Post, of *Ethics for Health Care Organizations: Theory, Case Studies, and Tools* (2001). He coedited, with Carol Levine and Nancy Dubler, *The Adolescent Alone,* a collection of essays, case studies, and guidelines relating to the care of unsupervised adolescents (1999). Blustein has published numerous articles and reviews in ethics and bioethics in leading scholarly journals and is a frequent speaker on issues in bioethics at regional and national meetings. In 2001 he was elected a fellow of the New York Academy of Medicine.

Judith Feder, Ph.D., is a professor and the dean of public policy at Georgetown University, in Washington, D.C. Under her leadership Georgetown's Public

Policy Institute draws on the university's academic excellence and the extraordinary resources of the nation's capital to train highly skilled and committed policy professionals for leadership positions in private firms; federal, state, and local government (including the District of Columbia); and nonprofit organizations. Feder is also a senior scholar at Georgetown's Institute of Health Care Research and Policy. She is one of the nation's leaders in health policy—particularly in efforts to understand and improve the nation's health insurance system. Feder has held leadership policy positions in both the Congress and the Executive Branch. She is a senior advisor to the Kaiser Family Foundation's Commission on Medicaid and the Uninsured; codirector, with Sheila Burke, of Kaiser's Incremental Health Reform Project and of Robert Wood Johnson's Long-Term Care project; a member of the board of the Academy of Health Services Research and Health Policy and the editorial boards of health policy journals; and a member of the National Academy of Public Administration and the National Academy of Social Insurance.

Gladys Gonzalaz-Ramos, M.S.W., Ph.D., is an associate professor at the New York University (NYU) School of Social Work and adjunct associate professor of neurology at the NYU Medical School. For more than twenty years she has been involved in program development, service delivery, research, and consultation in the mental health field. She has worked and published extensively in the area of services for the Latino population. For the past several years she has received foundation funding to study the needs of individuals and family caregivers affected by Parkinson disease. In collaboration with the National Parkinson Foundation, she is studying, on a national basis, the needs of underserved communities affected by Parkinson disease, with the goal of establishing systems of care which are responsive to the existing multiple needs of both patients and caregivers. In addition, Gonzalez-Ramos maintains a private practice in New York City.

David A. Gould, Ph.D., is a senior vice president for program of the United Hospital Fund of New York. He is responsible for the annual distribution of approximately six million dollars in philanthropic funds through the fund's discretionary grants in support of innovative health care projects and formula allocations reflecting charity care provided by member hospitals; for the management of its program development, policy analysis, and health services research staff; and for the direction of the fund's conference activities. Gould has directed the development of the fund's major initiatives, including palliative care, family caregiving, primary care development, and aging-in-place. In addition, he has served on a number of leadership commissions responsible for developing policy recommendations on a range of health care issues, including the Attorney General's Commission on Quality Care at the End of Life, the New York State Task Force on Long Term Care, the New York State Labor–Health Industry Task Force on Health Personnel, and the New York State Council on Home Care Services. He currently chairs the National Advisory Committee of the Center to Advance Palliative Care at the Mount Sinai School of Medicine. He has chaired the grant-making committee of the New York City AIDS Fund since its inception in 1988 and served on the board of Funders Concerned about AIDS.

Eileen Hanley, R.N., M.B.A., is the director of the Supportive Care Program and Manager for the Palliative Care Service at St. Vincent's Hospital Manhattan / Saint Vincent Catholic Medical Centers, New York City. A nurse with more than twenty-five years of acute care and community health experience in both direct care and administration, she has worked extensively with special-needs populations, including people living with HIV/AIDS, people with physical disabilities, and terminally ill persons. Hanley was the director of AIDS Services at the Visiting Nurse Service of New York (VNSNY), at the time the largest home care program for people with AIDS in the country. She was also the administrator of a large, multiple-site Medicare-certified hospice program for the VNSNY. Hanley is a member of the Board of Trustees of the Hospice and Palliative Care Association of New York State and is the chair of the association's Palliative Care Task Force. As the director of Clinical Services for Independence Care System, she helped to develop and implement a unique program of coordinated care for Medicaid-eligible individuals living with significant physical disabilities. She is also a member of the Regent's Advisory Council for the American College of HealthCare Executives for the New York region.

Maggie Hoffman is a cofounder and codirector of Project DOCC: Delivery of Chronic Care. Hoffman is the founder and facilitator of New Survivors, a peer support group for parents of children with chronic illness and/or disabilities. She is the founder and cochair of the Long Island Network for Families of Children with Special Healthcare Needs, a collaborative advocacy group composed of consumers and providers. Hoffman was the family-centered care specialist for the North Shore–Long Island Jewish Health System, New York. She coordinates the Project DOCC activities in partnership with the United Hospital Fund. She is currently working toward a degree in health care advocacy at Sarah Lawrence College and is the mother of Jacob, Rosie, and Molly (deceased).

Alexis Kuerbis, C.S.W., is the family therapist at the Mount Sinai Medical Center Alcohol and Other Drug Treatment Program, where she administers the Family Care Program and the on-site CASAWORKS for Families Project of the National Center on Addiction and Substance Abuse at Columbia University. She teaches courses on both alcoholism and bioethical issues at St. Joseph's College of New York, in Brooklyn. Kuerbis worked on the Families and Health Care Project at United Hospital Fund for four years, during which time she worked on the National Caregiving Survey Report and published a chapter in *Always on Call.* She continues to do freelance writing and research.

Carol Levine, M.A., directs the Families and Health Care Project of the United Hospital Fund, in New York City. This project focuses on developing partnerships between health care professionals and family caregivers who provide most of the long-term and chronic care to elderly, seriously ill, or disabled relatives. In 1998 she wrote a United Hospital Fund special report, *Rough Crossings: Family Caregivers' Odysseys through the Health Care System,* which explores patients' transitions between care settings and their impact on the family caregiver. She also directs the Orphan Project: Families and Children in the HIV Epidemic, which she founded in 1991. She was the director of the Citizens Commission on AIDS in New York City from 1987 to 1991. As a senior staff associate of The Hastings Center, she edited the *Hastings Center Report.* In 1993 she was awarded a MacArthur Foundation Fellowship for her work in AIDS policy and ethics. She has written several books and articles, including a "Sounding Board" essay in the *New England Journal of Medicine* entitled "The Loneliness of the Long-Term Care Giver" (May 20, 1999). She most recently edited *Always On Call: When Illness Turns Families into Caregivers,* 2d ed. (2004).

Jerome K. Lowenstein, M.D., is a professor of medicine and the chief of the Nephrology Division at the New York University Medical Center. He initiated in 1979 and continues to direct the program for Humanistic Aspects of Medical Education, which involves small-group meetings for third-year medical students during their clerkship in medicine and all of the medical house staff during their rotations through the medical intensive care unit and the AIDS units at Bellevue Hospital and Tisch Hospital. Since 1996 he has been responsible for the first-year patient narrative course. He is the author of *Acid and Basics: A Guide to Understanding Acid-Base Physiology* (1993) and *The Midnight Meal and Other Essays about Doctors, Patients, and Medicine* (1997). He is the editor for nonfiction of the newly created *Bellevue Literary Review*. Lowenstein received his M.D. degree from the New York University School of Medicine in 1957.

Mathy Mezey, R.N., Ed.D., is the Independence Foundation Professor of Nursing Education and the director of the John A. Hartford Foundation Institute for the Advancement of Geriatric Nursing Practice at New York University. She worked as a public health nurse and on medical and surgical units at Jacobi Hospital in the Bronx, New York, an acute-care facility of the New York City Health and Hospitals Corporation. Mezey taught at Lehman College of the City University of New York. For ten years she was a professor at the University of Pennsylvania School of Nursing, where she directed the geriatric nurse practitioner program and was the director of the Robert Wood Johnson Foundation Teaching Nursing Home Program. Her current research and writing focus is on ethical decision making about life-sustaining treatment. Mezey is exploring decision making by spouses of patients with Alzheimer disease and preparing guidelines to assist in decisions related to the transfer of patients between nursing homes and hospitals. She has written five books and more than fifty publications that focus on the nursing care of elderly individuals and on bioethical issues that affect decisions at the end of life.

Thomas H. Murray, Ph.D., is president of The Hastings Center, in Garrison, New York. He was formerly the director of the Center for Biomedical Ethics in the School of Medicine at Case Western Reserve University, where he was also the Susan E. Watson Professor of Bioethics. Murray's research interests cover a wide range of ethical issues in medicine and science, including genetics, children, organ donation, and health policy. He is a founding editor of the journal *Medical Humanities Review* and is on the editorial boards of *Human Gene Therapy; Politics and the Life Sciences; Cloning, Science, and Policy; Medscape Gen-*

eral Medicine; and *Teaching Ethics.* He is also editor, with Maxwell J. Mehlman, of the *Encyclopedia of Ethical, Legal and Policy Issues in Biotechnology* (2000). He served as a member of the U.S. Olympic Committee's Anti-Doping Committee, is currently a member of the Ethics and Education Committee of the World Anti-Doping Agency, and from 1996 to 2001 served as a presidential appointee to the National Bioethics Advisory Commission, for which he served as chair of the subcommittee on genetics. He served as a member of the Committee on Ethics of the American College of Obstetrics and Gynecology and is former chair of the Social Issues Committee of the American Society for Human Genetics. He is currently a member of the Ethics Committee of HUGO, the Human Genome Organization. He is past president of the Society for Health and Human Values and of the American Society for Bioethics and Humanities. He is the author of more than two hundred publications. His most recent books are *The Worth of a Child* and *Healthcare Ethics and Human Values: An Introductory Text with Readings and Case Studies,* which he edited with Bill Fulford and Donna Dickenson.

Judah L. Ronch, Ph.D., is the founder and executive clinical director of Life Span DevelopMental Systems, which for more than twenty-five years has created numerous innovative programs of clinical service, research, systems consultation, and organizational development to meet the mental health needs of aging people in various parts of the United States. Notable current activities include numerous culture change consultations in long-term care settings, nursing home program innovations in person-centered dementia care, work with the New York State Department of Health on dementia care practices in adult care facilities, and the Electronic Dementia Guide for Excellence (EDGE) program, an Internet-enabled system of tools and approaches designed to help nursing and assisted living facilities individualize and humanize care of residents with Alzheimer disease and related dementias. He maintains an active research program in the fields of innovative models of dementia care and culture change in long-term care. He is the former executive director of the Brookdale Center on Aging of Hunter College. Ronch's numerous publications include *Alzheimer's Disease: A Practical Guide for Families and Other Helpers* and *The Counseling Sourcebook: A Practical Reference on Contemporary Issues,* winner of the 1995 Catholic Press Association of the United States Book Award. He is the coeditor of the forthcoming books *Mental Wellness in Aging: Strength Based Approaches* and *Culture Change in Long-Term Care.*

Sheila M. Rothman, Ph.D., is a professor of public health in the Department of Sociomedical Sciences at Columbia University's Mailman School of Public Health, in New York City. She is also the deputy director of the Center for the Study of Society and Medicine at the Columbia College of Physicians and Surgeons. Her current research focuses on genetics, with a special interest in understanding the impact of new genetic knowledge on group identity. She is co–principal investigator, with David J. Rothman, on "The Genome Project and the Technologies of Enhancement" (National Institutes of Health), whose goal is to identify and analyze the challenges that genetic enhancements pose for U.S. health policy and social policy. She currently serves as a member of the Task Force on Human Genetics at the College of Physicians and Surgeons and chairs the Task Force on Genetics and Public Health at the Mailman School of Public Health. Rothman is also interested in the links between human rights and medicine. Together with David Rothman, she has published articles on how AIDS came to Romania and medical accountability in Zimbabwe in the *New York Review of Books*. Since 1995 she has been a member of the Bellagio Task Force on Securing Bodily Integrity for the Socially Disadvantaged: Strategies for Controlling the Traffic in Organs for Transplantation. She is the principal investigator of a multiple-site study that is analyzing patient and family decision making regarding organ donation in the United States.

Rick Surpin is the founder and president of Independence Care System (ICS), a nonprofit, Medicaid-managed, long-term care organization for adults with physical disabilities. ICS coordinates the care of a wide range of health and social services to enable people with significant disabilities, who are eligible for placement in a nursing home, to remain at home. He is also the founder and chair of two affiliated organizations that focus on creating high-quality jobs for paraprofessional health care workers and high-quality care for elderly persons and adults with physical disabilities: Cooperative Home Care Associates, a worker-owned home care agency in the South Bronx; and the Paraprofessional Healthcare Institute, a national nonprofit research and policy advocacy organization.

Foreword

Culture is a term we apply freely to explain the behavior and attitudes of people who think and act differently from ourselves. As health care professionals, we do not often think of culture as affecting our own actions and attitudes. Yet the authors in this stimulating book have done a great service in reflecting on their own and their colleagues' professional cultures and on the ways in which their patterns of behavior interact with the distinctive cultures of families as they deal with the challenges of illness and disability.

My perspective is that of a physician, embedded in a particular professional culture. Like the contributors to the book, I am not an anthropologist. If I were, I might be able, after extensive observation and analytical distance, to describe objectively the physician culture and its relationship to family caregiving. But I voluntarily sought a career in geriatrics and ethics, which has helped bring me close to family caregivers. Looking back, I can see that my experiences support the premise of this book.

In reaching a better understanding of how family caregivers interact with the health care system, we should not turn medicine into a monolith. We need to talk about the different cultures of medicine, its institutions, and how physicians' culture has evolved, especially in the last thirty years or so, and how it is still evolving. Nevertheless, it is fair to say that our dominant medical culture places a high value on cognitive and technical mastery, certainty, technology, scientific evidence, and hierarchy. Physicians are trained for mastery, and specialized skills are revered. These values, singly and in combination, often underlie conflicts between medicine and families. It is not that families do not value "good"—that is, technically proficient—doctoring. They do. But families' priorities, especially in chronic or terminal illness, are weighted toward actions that build or sustain relationships. When technical expertise has limits, communication, compassion, and consideration become even more paramount.

Certainty is related to mastery. Because physicians are expected to master a complex body of knowledge and skills, they want as much certainty as possible. Physicians become frustrated with patients and families who don't want as many tests as they would like to order and with managed care companies that refuse to pay for these tests. They will be reluctant to give a prognosis without certainty, but to share uncertainty is seen as admitting defeat. Yet, when patients and families ask for a prognosis, they often want reassurance, not necessarily a statistical probability. Physicians are too often ill equipped to give reassurance and, instead, give impersonal statistics.

Technology promotes certainty and mastery, but it also creates situations in which there is not as much therapeutic room to negotiate with the family. Fiber optics, for example, introduced a dramatic change; now inserting a feeding tube is no longer major surgery and can be done at the bedside. As a consequence, discussions about life-sustaining treatment occur in a different context of risks and benefits. Now family caregivers are making decisions about this procedure when it is technically less risky but ethically still challenging. Because the procedure is easily done, physicians may not seize the opportunity to discuss with the family the momentous decision at hand—to allow a natural death or to prolong life, with its inevitable medical complications and suffering—which may not be consistent with the patient's values.

While the formal curriculum of medical education does not prepare physicians to work well with families, the informal curriculum of residency training teaches the wrong lessons. Indoctrination into the physician culture begins early. When I was a medical student, doing a rotation in neurology at Massachusetts General Hospital, a resident asked me to do a lumbar puncture. (Although I had never performed this procedure before, the resident didn't come into the patient's room with me. I was supposed to call if I got into trouble.) The patient had wet the bed, and I thought I should change the sheets before doing the puncture. The resident found me changing the bed and chastised me for engaging in such "unprofessional" behavior. Changing linens, I learned, was a nurse's or aide's job, not a physician's. The culture of medicine is transmitted not just through the formal curriculum but even more intensely through on-the-job experiences.

Later, when I was a fellow in geriatric medicine in Portland, I overheard a conversation about a patient between a resident and an intern, in which the resident complained, "Her family is terrible—they're *here* all the time." Because the family, in their view, was in the way, it was harder for the resident and intern to accomplish their technical goals. Of course, from the patient's and family's view, "being there" was an essential manifestation of their long-standing affection and fidelity.

The role models for residents and students are all too often physicians who, distinguished though they may be in the technical aspects of medicine, show a lack of respect toward the students, residents, patients, and families. Not surprisingly, then, physicians-in-training exposed to this model often become inattentive to small courtesies and ordinary politeness. A study of patient satisfaction showed that the most important variable that led to a positive attitude was whether the physician introduced him- or herself to the patient. What is it about the physician culture that leads to this suspension of the ordinary rules of behavior and ultimately to the physician and family seeing each other as problems?

Especially in geriatrics, families may be seen as negligent (accused of elder abuse or "granny dumping") if they don't follow through with the demands of medicine. Meanwhile, families are concerned about undertreatment, overtreatment, and medical mistakes. They are suspicious of the cost-cutting financial environment that pervades health care today.

Physicians nod in deference to patient and family decision making but expect families to "decide" what we want them to decide. We ask families to provide technical medical care at home, for which they are inadequately trained before the patient is discharged from the hospital. Then we call them "non-compliant" if they fail to follow the complex regimens we have devised.

In their training physicians experience a highly rigid hierarchy: student, resident, fellow, professor, and great professor. Hierarchy is embedded in every aspect of medical practice and training. There are good reasons for this; it is essential to know who is in charge in emergencies. But sometimes decision making should be more collaborative, and here the hierarchical model is a barrier. The continual evolution of medicine also can frustrate families. On the one hand, with the ascendancy of medical "teams," family caregivers are not sure who is in charge. On the other hand, the hospitalist movement poses a different challenge. In this increasingly prevalent practice the patient's primary care doctor, who knows the patient and family best, does not provide hospital care. The hospital physician is more readily available for family discussions, however, than the primary care doctor would be.

Physicians are neither well trained nor professionally supported in dealing with the dynamics of family culture. As with medicine, hierarchy is breaking

down in the family. We don't know for sure who will be the family negotia-
tor when a decision must be made for an incompetent patient. Physicians
aren't trained to deal with the patient's and family's complex social and economic problems, and they look to nurses and social workers as the interface
between the family and the rest of the medical world. Yet nurses' and social
workers' roles—indeed, their very availability—are changing in hospitals as
well, and families may be perplexed and lost in the shuffle.

Physicians are trained to think that their responsibilities are to individual
patients. This is part of the Hippocratic ethic and the legal assumption of
fiduciary responsibility. Medical ethics focuses on responsibilities to individual patients, not families. This creates dilemmas; for example, in diagnoses
of early Alzheimer disease, should a physician tell the family or the patient first? What is the physician's responsibility to anyone other than the
patient?

Family medicine challenges this notion of the individual as the only object
of physician responsibility. Family medicine was developed in the 1960s to
address needs that medicine was not meeting in communities. Rather than
specialize in technical or intellectual skills or a particular age group, family
medicine followed a different model with different cultural characteristics:
the family is the unit of care, not the individual. The impact of illness of one
family member is assumed to affect the others. This model assumes a relationship and responsibility to the whole family and challenges physicians to
behave differently.

Other, more recent changes in the culture of medicine present new opportunities. In general we are developing a broader concern about population
health (health maintenance versus disease treatment). Genetics will enable
more powerful prevention models. With enrolled populations in managed
care, more may be done in schools and other less medical settings. If this is
true, medicine is using an ethic of fundamental utilitarianism, rather than
maximizing goods for single patients. This shift will dramatically change
many aspects of the medical culture.

Yet, although the advent of managed care can have a positive impact on
the culture of medicine, the backlash by both physicians and individuals
threatens many positive bonds. The government is creating new laws and regulations to protect consumers, and physicians and patients are suspicious
about decision making by managed care organizations. They believe that the
incentives are financial, rather than based on quality of care. But the system
of decisions driven by hidden financial incentives creates a new divide be-

tween the physician and a patient and his or her family which makes deliberative, shared decision making even more difficult.

Several authors in the book point out areas of common ground between health care professionals and family caregivers. We need to build on our shared values, seeking to provide compassionate health care in a system that is dominated by the values of mastery, certainty, technology, and hierarchy. We need to look at the bigger picture in which cultures and institutions have the power to shape individuals' attitudes and behavior.

Like the health care system and families, medical education is also changing, stimulated by public and professional concern about quality of care and leadership by accreditation and certification bodies. In 2002 the Accreditation Council of Graduate Medical Education instituted a new requirement that all residency training programs (no matter what specialty) require physicians to demonstrate their graduate competency in six areas: medical knowledge, patient care, communication skills, professionalism, practice improvement, and systems-based practice. While medical knowledge and patient care are standard and time-honored expectations, the other four competencies will stretch training programs as they discover how to teach and evaluate these skills. Professionalism and communication skills are directly related to caregiver concerns. Performance improvement and systems-based practice force recognition of the requirement for public accountability and professional responsibility to evaluate the quality of one's own practice, using interdisciplinary perspectives and patient-oriented outcome measures.

Certifying boards that measure and set physician performance standards in the major specialties have accepted the need to embrace these kinds of competencies—especially professionalism and quality improvement—in their own evaluation processes. These trends will have a major influence on education and training programs and will stimulate faculty to learn these approaches so that they can effectively teach students. Practicing physicians will want to demonstrate their continuing competency to maintain certification. Patients and family caregivers should come to expect more from us and to become active participants at all levels in the constructive feedback that is central to the quality improvement process.

Christine K. Cassel, M.D., M.A.C.P.
President and Chief Executive Officer,
American Board of Internal Medicine and
ABIM Foundation

Preface

This book began, as so many interesting projects do, as a casual observation after a series of meetings. When the United Hospital Fund's Families and Health Care Project was launched in 1996, we convened a number of meetings with health care professionals from several disciplines and cultural and ethnic backgrounds to discuss family caregiving. We also convened focus groups of caregivers to learn more about their experiences with health care professionals. Although the stated topic of one professionals' meeting was to explore how their origins as Latinos or African Americans affected their perceptions of family, the conversation invariably turned toward the way they, as professionals, responded to family concerns and the way the "culture" of their institution dictated much of their response. Family members, for their part, saw health professionals as representatives of an arcane and byzantine world, where ordinary rules of discourse and behavior were suspended. It was almost as if, we observed, families and health care professionals come from different cultures.

What might that mean? We decided to explore the idea further, and, supported by the United Hospital Fund's grant-making capacity as well as its research and analytical strengths, we collaborated with The Hastings Center, well-known for its ability to bring together diverse working groups to discuss ethical issues in health care. Over the course of a year and a half, from late 1999 to 2001, the center organized two day-and-a-half-long meetings. Some members of the working group subsequently presented the project findings at a United Hospital Fund conference and discussed the project with the Families and Health Care Advisory Committee and grantees of the Family Caregiving Initiative. This book has evolved from that collaboration.

The authors in this book, all members of the working group, approach the basic theme of caregiving as seen from the perspective of families, professionals, and policy makers. Although each family caregiver's experience is unique, there are some common themes. Part 1, which considers "Perspectives on

Family Caregiving," begins with a chapter by David A. Gould in which he summarizes the national results of a random telephone survey of caregivers conducted by the Harvard School of Public Health, the Visiting Nurse Service of New York, and the United Hospital Fund. He provides a rich demographic portrait of the nation's family caregivers, the tasks they undertake, and the challenges they face. Of particular importance is the survey's documentation of the lack of coordination between family caregivers and the formal health care system. These data reveal that family caregivers are poorly prepared to take on their daunting, frequently medicalized tasks and that they have significant unmet needs.

The next two chapters turn from data to personal narratives. Gladys Gonzalez-Ramos recounts the searing experience of coping with her mother's Parkinson disease and her father's growing inability to accept the incapacity of his beloved wife. Although she is a professor of social work, Gonzalez-Ramos learned how ill prepared she was to manage her parents' interactions with the health care system. Although this story is extreme in its outcome, the basic problem of the health care system's fragmentation and narrow medical focus is common. Gonzalez-Ramos is Cuban-American; her parents' final struggle is all the more poignant because of their earlier adjustment to the unfamiliar American culture. In this case cultural difference in the more common sense of language and ethnicity added to the family's distress. Gonzalez-Ramos's emphasis on the memories and idealizations of the homeland which occur when illness strikes a family is surely applicable to people from many other immigrant backgrounds.

Jerome K. Lowenstein, a nephrologist, presents a vignette from his own experience dealing with patients and family members. His patient was discovered to have metastatic cancer, and Lowenstein was preparing to deliver the grim news, when the patient's wife pleaded with him to withhold the diagnosis. In time Lowenstein came to believe that his "need" to deliver the truth, as the current medical culture dictates, did not automatically trump the family's understanding of its own needs and welfare. "Patients," he writes, "experience *illness* as a unique, personal, idiosyncratic event. Physicians understand *disease*."

The second part, "Home Care Past and Present," makes clear the roots of this disjunction. Sheila M. Rothman takes us back to nineteenth-century New England, when nearly all medical care was family care. But, as she shows with contemporary data and narratives, family care was not just the responsibility of a few individuals but of whole communities. The women in these communities, whatever their marital status, provided care to kin and neighbors, even traveling long distances to do so. Since many of the ill were suffering from tuberculosis, this care could be long and drawn-out. As long as it was believed that tuberculosis was noncontagious and affected all social classes, home care was the main caretaking system. The introduction of the germ theory, the rise of tuberculosis in urban slums, and the growth of institutional placement for the afflicted began to take medical care out of the home and into special institutions, where professionals held sway. Families were relegated to the sidelines. Rothman observes that, because of economic forces and the decline of institutions, family care is once again dominant, but today's families lack the earlier support of community and culture.

Mathy Mezey takes the story to the next phase. The private-duty nurse of the late nineteenth and early twentieth centuries, employed mainly by well-to-do families, was neither a full professional nor a domestic servant. In the public health realm nurses helped ill patients in poor communities and taught their families how to provide care. As hospitals grew more powerful and nursing became professionalized, home care nursing lost prestige. And more recently, with the introduction of high-technology hospital care, nurses perceived high-tech care as the best way to use their scientific knowledge and clinical skills. Nursing educators teach that the nurse's role encompasses the family, but in practice nurses are often too burdened by other responsibilities to do very much training or communication. Mezey does, however, point to some promising innovations in service provision as hopeful signs.

Rick Surpin and Eileen Hanley see the passage of Medicare and Medicaid in 1965 as a defining moment in home care. From then on these programs, in which long-term or chronic care was never an important part of the original drafters' plan, directed the way in which home care was delivered by the thousands of agencies that grew up to provide the funded services. Under Medicare nursing care was defined not by the profession but by regulators as "skilled" but "intermittent" and "part-time" care. A new job category—the home care aide—was created to provide the "unskilled" part of the service. Surpin and Hanley describe the work arrangements of home care aides and the way in which they are both "like family" and "part of the system." They offer useful advice about assessing home care situations so that tensions between families and aides, and between aides and their supervising nurses, might be eased. They, too, see some hopeful signs in recent innovative projects.

Part 3, "The Societal Context," looks at two very different cultures. Judith Feder and Carol Levine judiciously describe the policy culture that sets the rules and regulations for Medicare and, by extension, most of third-party payer policies regarding home care. One fundamental assumption is that the individual, not the family, is the sole beneficiary. Family caregivers are not entitled to anything beyond what they might receive as beneficiaries themselves. Feder and Levine point out that policy makers look at programs from the point of view of the entire population of potentially eligible individuals, not at the impact on specific individuals or families. Public funding brings with it the obligation to use resources sparingly and to set up systems of eligibility and accountability which are easily monitored and controlled. The kinds of restrictions which family caregivers find so frustrating (such as the "homebound rule" for Medicare and the distinction between skilled and unskilled care) are, from a policy view, simply ways to limit care to the most vulnerable. If restrictions are loosened, policy makers fear an uncontrollable flood of applicants and expenses. Underlying this view is the assumption that families *ought* to provide care and that government (or insurance companies) should only step in when there is no family or when families do not, for whatever reason, provide the needed care.

The second chapter in Part 3 looks at popular culture, specifically the movies, in portraying family caregivers in ways that marginalize, idealize, demonize, eroticize, and occasionally realistically enact their lives. Carol Levine and Alexis Kuerbis illustrate each of these genres. They argue that the images in these films are not just entertainment but are important in shaping popular views about family caregiving. How caregivers are presented lends support to public policy makers' and professionals' particular assumptions and values; such images may also give caregivers unrealistic standards against which to measure their own feelings and actions.

Although some of the authors in earlier sections make recommendations for change, the final part, "Bridging the Gap among Cultures," looks specifically at current and future efforts to emphasize the shared values and minimize the tensions. Jeffrey Blustein asserts that core physician and family values do, in fact, have a lot in common, despite the tensions that exist. He sees the differences as largely due to the "corrupting influence of socially pervasive values that shape but are not confined to medicine." He envisions a partnership between families and professionals, not a blurring of their respective roles, which occurs when professionals try to fill the void caused by absent or inadequate family members or when they attempt to provide on-going care to their own family members. He, like several other authors, points to hospice as an example of a care system that values and practices collaboration and family involvement. The philosophy of hospice, he suggests, should be extended to other arenas of care.

Maggie Hoffman and Donna Jean Appell describe one successful attempt to bridge the gap. As parents of chronically ill and disabled children and founders of Project DOCC (Delivery of Chronic Care), they have developed a parent-directed program in which parents present pediatric grand rounds, bring pediatric residents into the home to see how families with disabled children really live, and work with medical educators to build collaborative relationships.

Finally, Judah L. Ronch analyzes the reasons that institutions (primarily hospitals and long-term care facilities) do not typically support the attitudes and behaviors that bring a sense of accomplishment to workers and satisfaction to patients and family members. Institutional care is rooted in "standards and practices designed to promote the medical well-being of patients." Although certainly necessary, this care lacks adequate ways to meet the human needs of patients, family members, and workers. He proposes that the process of changing the culture of institutions begin by "identifying where all the key stakeholders share common motivation and by demonstrating where the current culture keeps each of them from realizing their higher aspirations." These relationships can then be reframed from being conflict based and competitive to being collaborative. He especially looks to "positive deviants"—the people who on their own find creative ways to "humanize the culture"—as leaders of change.

A concluding chapter, by the editors, brings together the main themes and offers some further reflections on ways to bridge the culture gap.

In sum, the authors in this volume bring to life a complex but still evolving picture of the cultures of caregiving. Our goal, as coeditors and codirectors of the project that began this exploration, is to stimulate discussion and reflection on these themes. As family caregivers are challenged to assume more and more difficult responsibilities for an aging population, it is time for all the actors in this drama to think clearly about the values that shape their actions. A health care system built on a culture that equally values technical skill and compassionate care must rethink the current ways it treats family caregivers. It is no longer justifiable to dismiss family caregivers as troublesome exten-

sions of the patient or to exploit them as free labor. The power of the culture
of families must stimulate change.

In addition to the authors in this volume, we would like to acknowledge
the thoughtful and insightful participation of other members of the working
group and invited guests at the meetings convened by the United Hospital
Fund and The Hastings Center (their affiliations are listed for identification
only): John Arras, University of Virginia; Andrew Billingsley, Columbia, S.C.;
Christine Cassel, American Board of Internal Medicine; Henry Chung, Pfizer,
Inc; Alan Fleischman, New York Academy of Medicine; Ruby H. Greene, RHG
Associates; Eva Feder Kittay, State University of New York–Stony Brook; Kenny
Kwong, Chinatown Health Clinic, New York City; Harry R. Moody, Institute
for Human Values in Aging; Carmen Ortiz-Neu, New York–Presbyterian Hospitals; Rachel Pruchno, Boston College; and Rabbi Gerald Wolpe, Philadelphia. In addition, several staff members of The Hastings Center and the
United Hospital Fund also attended the meetings. We would particularly like
to thank Debbie Halper and Susan Hopper of the fund and Erik Parens of the
center for their contributions. Jodi Fernandes at the center and Alexis Kuerbis
of the fund expertly organized the logistics of the meetings. Shoshana
Vasheetz and Helen Maio at the fund efficiently prepared the manuscript for
publication. For their guidance in preparing this volume, we would like to
thank copyeditor Elizabeth Gratch and Wendy Harris and Clare Lochary at
the Johns Hopkins University Press.

The Cultures of Caregiving

Caregiving as a Family Affair

A New Perspective on Cultural Diversity

Carol Levine and Thomas H. Murray

Health care is, among many other things, a series of dramas, some tragic, some comic, some inspiring, some dismaying, and most utterly ordinary. Even the most mundane story, however, is meaningful to the actors. While a great deal of attention has been understandably devoted to the main characters—physicians and patients—and the relationship between them others also play significant roles onstage and off. Each actor brings a special interpretation to the scene, and each plays the role not only by reading the lines but also by bringing his or her whole worldview to the enactment.

This book explores that theme in some of its many variations. The basic premise is this: *Families, health care professionals, and health policy makers and administrators have distinctive cultures—ways of viewing the world—which affect their priorities and actions in the care of an elderly or ill person.* Culture in this sense includes but goes beyond ethnicity, religion, or language; it encompasses a shared understanding of a way of life which encompasses principles, values, attitudes, and behaviors based on membership in a group, whether that is family, professional discipline, institution, or agency. This concept, we believe, illuminates many of the tensions and conflicts that occur in health care, especially those that involve family caregivers. Although there are common elements and points of congruence among these cultures, as several authors point out, we focus here on the areas of divergence. It is in this area that the trouble lies and where we need fresh approaches.

To begin this exploration, consider the following scene, fictional but reality based, from the points of view of the actors.* We shall return to it later.

Outside the Patient's hospital room, 7:30 A.M. **The doctor reviews the case in his mind.**

The Doctor: My patient is a seventy-eight-year-old-female with a history of heart disease. She is in the hospital because she fell at home during a dizzy spell and broke her hip. The patient's surgery went well. She has not responded as well, however, to the rehabilitation process. The physical therapist's report indicates that the Patient has been willing to do exercises but has not shown significant gait stability. Although there was no documented note indicating the need for further inpatient treatment, the physical therapist told the discharge planner and me that the Patient would benefit from a few more inpatient days.

The cardiologist has seen the Patient and recommended increasing the dose of her antiarrhythmic medication and sees no reason why she cannot be followed as an outpatient to assess her response. He has no opposition to discharge today, especially after I told him that the daughter is very involved and can monitor her symptoms. I asked a pulmonologist to stop by and evaluate her because the physical therapist says she gets short of breath easily. She ordered pulmonary function tests and a chest X ray, but I doubt that there's anything going on. The chest X ray is clear, but the other test results won't be available until tomorrow.

The social worker reporting to the discharge planner would like more time to plan for home visitation services, but the discharge planner notes that the Patient belongs to a Medicare HMO, and it feels that the Patient is stable and can be discharged. The Medicare HMO states that it will have a nurse visit the Patient and determine what additional services might be necessary.

*We are grateful to Henry Chung, M.D., who supplied the medical details of this scenario and played the role of The Doctor in a United Hospital Fund conference on May 9, 2000. Alexis Kuerbis and Gladys Gonzalez-Ramos, along with the editors, also took part in this and another reading.

In an ideal world I would keep the Patient in the hospital for a few more days, but she's been begging to leave every time I visit her. I don't have any unresolved medical issues. I can manage this case very well on an outpatient basis. Besides, I understand the daughter comes to visit regularly. She can hold the fort until I see the Patient in one week. Let's push for discharge today.

Inside the hospital room the Caregiver also reviews the situation.
The Caregiver: The Patient is my mother. She has been living alone since my father died four years ago. I was worried that something like this would happen because I don't think she takes her heart medication all the time. She wants to be independent, but she really can't manage by herself anymore. Sometimes she seems like her old self—funny, stubborn, and involved with the members of her senior club—and sometimes she seems totally distant and forgetful. Her apartment is pretty messy, and this is a woman who never left a floor unscrubbed or a dish unwashed. But, every time I offer to help her or send in a cleaning service, she gets very insulted. I really can't afford to help her much financially, but she won't even accept the little I can offer.

My sister and my brother are concerned about her, but they don't live here. When they do see her, and it's always at my house, she manages to pull herself together for their benefit. So, they think she's fine, but I know she's not. At least she'll be here in the hospital for a few more days until she's stronger and can walk.

I got here early this morning to talk to the Doctor. He's never here when I am. I hope he comes soon because I have to get to work. I've missed three days already this week, and I can't come right after work because I have a conference with Tommy's teacher. And I haven't had time to take care of anything at home.

The Doctor enters, followed by several young people in white coats.
The Doctor (heartily): Good morning, Mrs. A. I have good news for you. Your blood pressure is stable, and your hip is healing very nicely. You can definitely go home today!

The Patient (weakly): Oh, doctor, thank you. I can't wait to be in my own bed and eat what I like. This hospital food is terrible.

The Doctor: Well, you're going to have to stay on your special diet, no salt, low fat. I'm sure your daughter here will prepare your meals so that they follow the diet and taste good. And I'm going to increase the dose of your heart medicine. I don't want you to fall again. (*To the Caregiver*) I'd like to see Mother in about a week, so make an appointment with my office. (*To the Patient*) Someone will be by a little later with the paperwork, and then you're out of here!

The Caregiver: But, Doctor, my mother hasn't even been able to walk alone. Is it safe for her to go home?

The Doctor: She'll do fine. You can help her get to the bathroom. And make sure she doesn't stay in bed all day. She should be walking as much as possible.

The Caregiver: But my mother lives alone. Won't she need help?

The Doctor's beeper goes off. He looks at it and says hurriedly: Doesn't she live with you? Well, can she stay with you for a few weeks? If you don't want to do it, speak to the social worker on the floor. She'll find out if your mother is eligible for any home care. I'm sure we can work something out.

The Patient: I can manage on my own! I don't want any strangers in my house.

The Caregiver: (*To the Patient*) Now, Mother, don't get excited. We'll talk about that later. (*To the Doctor*) And why are you increasing the dose of her heart medicine? Are there any side effects?

The Doctor: She's been on this medication before—there's really nothing to worry about. Of course, if something seems wrong to you, call me right away.

The Caregiver (persisting): The doctor who stopped by yesterday seemed concerned about her breathing. She ordered some tests.

The Doctor: Well, we don't have the results yet. I'll try to follow up with you next week. Just in case, you should have her get another chest X ray before bringing her to see me. The social worker can set that up for you.

The Caregiver (looking at her mother): Oh, no! Mom, are you going to throw up? Are you okay? Where's the basin? Somebody help me!

The Doctor: Call the nurse. (*Leaving the room*) I have to answer the page. See you both in a week. I'm sure Mother will feel much better at home.

The Patient: What a nice man! I'm sorry I threw up, but I'm so happy I'm going home.

The Caregiver: Yes, Mom. I'm glad you're going home too. (*To herself*) How am I ever going to manage this?

A Different Perspective on Cultural Diversity

Now let's change the scene. Four families are seated in a nursing home (or hospital or agency) waiting room. They are speaking quietly, but there is an air of anxiety in the room. If you could listen in, you would hear four different languages, including varieties of English. They are from different ethnic groups: white, Asian American, African American, and Latino.

One large group is multigenerational; the teenagers hold their own conversations, all the while attentive to the needs of the elderly woman who seems to be their grandmother or perhaps their great-grandmother. Another group is made up of just two people, an elderly couple who seem to be married, but they might be brother and sister. The third group includes an elderly man and his adult daughters and their husbands. Three women make up the fourth group. The members of these groups have different styles of dress. Some are obviously more prosperous than others. Some wear religious symbols as pendants or pins.

What is the most distinctive characteristic of these families? Someone coming into the room might say that it's their language, their ethnicity, their social and economic class, or their religion. All these factors are important, of course, but what is often missed is that the characteristic that distinguishes these individuals from the professionals they encounter in the formal health care and social service system is that they are *families*. As people tied to one another through blood, marriage, or shared commitment, their priorities and values differ in some significant ways from those of the professionals with whom they will now begin to interact.

Nearly all the multiple versions of "caregiver burden scales" focus on the caregiver's stress that results from either the caregiver's lack of social support or the relationship with the care recipient. The "Caregiver Hassle Scale," despite its name, deals only with hassles that occur between caregiver and care recipient (Kinney and Stephens 1989). There is hardly a mention of one of the major stressors: unsatisfactory relationships with agents of the health care system, whether they are doctors, nurses, social workers, hospital or nursing home administrators, or insurance personnel.

Although health care professionals and family caregivers have the same broad goals for a patient/relative, as we have noted, the relationship between them is often strained and sometimes hostile (Levine and Zuckerman 1999). Why is this so? Usually, the answer from professionals is that a particular family is "dysfunctional" or that they "don't understand" the prognosis, the treatment, or whatever has become the issue of the moment. Families are criticized when they are too involved and when they are not involved enough. For their part families may describe a particular doctor or nurse as "cold," "uncaring," or "uncommunicative" and a social worker as "only interested in getting my father out of the hospital." But placing all the blame on individuals or personality conflicts misses a larger point.

Families and professionals have different assumptions, values, attitudes, and behaviors—in other words, they have different "cultures." The "cultural divide" between families and health professionals is the central focus of this book. But we can speak of cultural differences in other ways that also are relevant to home caregiving.

"Cultural diversity" has come to be equated with immigrant or minority families, yet all cultures, new and old, minority and majority, have special characteristics. Within each culture every family has its own blend of group and personal characteristics developed over time and generations through their shared history. And within each family different individuals have unique sets of beliefs, aspirations, strengths, and limitations.

Just as we now recognize that simplistic perceptions of what a person from a particular culture believes or would choose are outmoded, it is important to bring that same depth of understanding to family cultures. The early and innovative enthusiasm for bringing awareness of cultural diversity into professional training and practice at times risked stereotyping individuals according to dominant and sometimes cast-off attitudes and behaviors.

Cultures change. Sometimes this is rapid, at other times very slow. Cultures that do not adapt to changing physical, social, and economic environments risk their future viability. While "family" is an important part of every culture, the variants are many and rich. Think, for example, of blended families, gay and lesbian partnerships, multigenerational families, newly immigrant families, non-English-speaking families, adoptive families, single parent–headed households, and more. "Cultural competence"—the ideal to which all health care professionals should aspire—should include the ability to explore and respond appropriately to these diverse relationships without having preconceived ideas about them. This is especially critical in long-term care, which strains many families' cohesion and resources and which often brings health professionals onto the family's own turf, the home.

Despite their many differences, families, as fundamental units of society, are characterized by certain values, which are manifested in family caregiving, whether it takes place in the home or in a facility. Some of the primary values inherent in family caregiving are the importance of relationships established by blood, marriage, or commitment; a shared history, often involving several generations; except in extreme cases, the absence of public oversight or involvement; emotional rather than professional or financial rewards; moral rather than legal obligations; mutual expectations of support; flexible support structures; privacy of decision making; and family rather than individual autonomy. Except in a few cases, family members are not paid for their labor. Unlike professionals, who have a broad knowledge base but know a particular patient or client only in the context of his or her presenting problem, families know a great deal about all aspects of the person's life and history but not very much about the specific problem or issue. They are both experts but in different ways.

Some patterns do transcend different ethnicity, religion, and other cultural factors. The obligation of families to care for their ill and elderly members appears to be deep in every tradition, but the implementation may be difficult and unsupported because of contemporary circumstances. One example is the changing role of women, even in traditional families. Another is intergenerational or acculturation differences. In these cases family caregivers experience dissonance not only with the formal structure but also with their own tradition. Professionals, and caregivers themselves, may assume that support will come from the family and community, but the reality may be quite different.

In contrast to family culture, the U.S. health care system today is dominated by the culture of Western medicine: the primary values are scientific, evidence-based data; legal, regulatory, and professional oversight; efficiency; objectivity; consistency; confidentiality of medical information; technological solutions; hierarchical organizations; and individual patient autonomy. Professionals have special knowledge of a range of pertinent issues. They are trained to understand how a specific person fits within the larger set of people having similar problems and to devise solutions based on that knowledge.

Professional care providers (such as doctors, nurses, and social workers) get financial rewards and recognition, have professional associations, and gain community standing. Of course, not all professionals obtain these rewards in equal measure. The status of paraprofessionals—the indispensable home health aides and Certified Nursing Assistants (CNAs)—lies between families and professionals. Home health aides work in the private domain of family life, but their jobs are directed and controlled by a hierarchy of professional interests. CNAs have the most direct and prolonged contact with nursing home residents, but they, too, are supervised and regulated by professional and governmental agents.

Within both the broad cultures of health care and family there are, of course, many distinctions. In medicine cultures vary by specialty, institutional mission, and leadership; training and socialization; type of population served; and the personal background of professionals. Nurses and social workers have different cultures, but both value personal communication and building relationships. In family caregiving, families differ by structure, ethnic background, socioeconomic class, religion, degree of collaboration or conflict, and stages of life course, among other factors.

Professionals as Family Members

Professionals also come from families, many of them similar to the families they serve in their agencies or institutions. Having a common background or shared experience can certainly strengthen a professional's ability to understand a family's values and to communicate with them sensitively. Many families are more trusting of a professional who "speaks their language," whether that is literal or metaphorical.

A professional's family background and experience, however, can also be a barrier. Unexamined assumptions—even prejudices—about what family members "should" do may hinder an objective assessment of the situation. Gender roles are particularly sensitive in this regard. Based on their own family history or community standards, professionals can subtly or not so subtly express their opinion that a wife should quit her job to take care of her ill husband or that a daughter should bring her mother to live with her. It is not uncommon to hear professionals describing their culture as "valuing elders" when discussing a patient's family member who, in their view, is failing to take responsibility for an elder. The family member may be a person from their own culture, who is seen as not living up to (often idealized) community standards, or a person from another culture that is seen as inferior to one's own in this regard. Although pride in one's culture is admirable and can provide a moral anchor, it is important for professionals to refrain from imposing their own values and experiences on their clients and patients.

The most significant factor that comes between professionals and families, however, is most likely the professional role itself. Acting as a professional social worker, physician, or nurse, one knows and fulfills the routines, rules, and behaviors that reflect one's training and mark one's status. When a professional is put into the role of family caregiver, however, he or she often finds the situation as stressful, unpredictable, and frustrating as lay family members do. A recent study of physicians whose fathers had been ill found that "the physicians expressed concern about the care their fathers received, believing that the system does not operate the way it should" (Chen, Rhodes, and Green 2001). One physician said, "The system really didn't give me someone who I could talk to, who would understand me, understand our family, and understand the issues" (763). All of a sudden professional training and know-how vanish, and all the inadequacies and uncertainties of the fragmented, discontinuous health care system loom large. Sometimes these personal experiences alter for the better the professional's outlook and behavior in dealing with patients and families. Yet training and habit are powerful influences resisting change.

Professionals are also subject to societal and cultural influences beyond their own discipline. If there is a gap between professionals and families, there is another gap that is arguably even deeper—between professionals (and, to the degree their views are congruent, families) and policy makers and administrators. In the evolving health care economy professional values have been forced to adapt to the demands of the marketplace in health care, which is governed by a corporate or bureaucratic culture. While some of these strictures have been valuable in reducing waste and promoting consistency, there is an inevitable tension between the primary professional value of serving individuals and families and the economic and institutional requirements to serve larger entities, including other beneficiaries or health care group members, taxpayers, and stockholders. Some of the most important actors in our health care dramas are offstage, directing the action but hidden from view.

Text and Subtext

Let us return to the scene that began this chapter and look at the interactions from the point of view of each actor's culture.

The subtext from the Doctor's view

The Doctor's primary loyalty is to his patient. He believes that, from a strictly medical viewpoint, she can go home. The Patient has no more acute care medical needs, and the Doctor is also keenly aware of the hospital's pressures to discharge such patients. He is part of a system with clear constraints and professional relationships and does not want to be singled out at the next departmental meeting as someone who isn't following discharge guidelines. The pulmonologist argued that the Patient should stay until the test results are evaluated, but the Doctor does not think this is necessary. If the Doctor were alone in the room when the Patient vomited, he might have helped the daughter, but he wants the young residents to understand that this is not what physicians are supposed to do. He believes that the "social" aspects of his patient's care are not in his jurisdiction; he does not want to open a Pandora's box. He has never seen his patient's home and knows little about her family life. He assumes that the Daughter, who has been a faithful visitor, will manage everything.

The subtext from the Caregiver's view

The Caregiver is experiencing different, conflicting tensions. She is torn between her mother's desire to go home and her worry that she cannot provide the help her mother will need. She also feels that she is getting mixed messages from the Doctor. On the one hand, the Doctor is discharging her mother, but he's also increasing the medication, the effects of which have to be monitored. Although the Doctor says there is nothing to worry about, he suggests that her mother stay with her for a few weeks. The Caregiver wants to be a good daughter and do whatever is necessary to take care of her mother, but she worries that she's neglecting her husband, children, and job. She doesn't see how she can have her mother come and stay with them. She feels guilty about even bringing up her own concerns about her job and family, and so she focuses on the medical implications of bringing her mother home. She has not met the social worker on the floor, and the nursing staff has changed from shift to shift. There is no one for her to talk to about her concerns. She, too, is part of a system—a family system that includes her siblings, her husband, and her own children. She knows that her sister and brother will not be able to help out because they don't live nearby. She is afraid they will criticize her for any problems that arise.

The subtext from the Patient's view

The Patient wants to go home. She minimizes her dependence, which has been increasing. She believes that it is not only best for her but also easier for her daughter to be in her own home. She sees the Doctor as her ally and advocate. Because her daughter doesn't complain, she is not really aware of the time, expense, and stress the illness has caused. She does not like the idea of "strangers" coming into her home, partly out of fear but also because she does not want them to think badly of the current state of her housekeeping, which has deteriorated. She is trying desperately to keep up a good front and maintain a sense of her own autonomy.

The subtext from a policy maker's view

From the point of view of hospital administrators and payers, hospital stays should be minimized. Hospital stays are expensive and subject the patient to iatrogenic risks from infection and other sources. Patients who do not need the level of acute care provided in a hospital are better off at home and usually want to be there anyway. Additional necessary follow-up care can be provided on an outpatient basis. Home care is primarily a family responsibility, although some short-term additional support may be necessary for the transition. From all points of view—patient safety and satisfaction, cost containment, judicious use of resources—this patient should be discharged. The hospital's scarce resources can be better used for another patient with more urgent medical needs.

All the actors are playing roles for which their culture has ably prepared them. If we were to carry the scenario further and involve the nurse and social worker, they too would act in accord with their professional responsibilities, whatever they might personally feel about the discharge plan. The doctor has approved the discharge; it is up to them to see that it occurs as successfully as possible. The nurse may recognize the daughter's distress but only has time to give her information about the medications and potential side effects. The social worker can refer the patient to a home care agency for evaluation and possible services, but there her responsibility ends. And, as we shall see in succeeding chapters, the home care team, when it finally arrives on the scene, has its own culture as well as regulatory and financial limitations.

Conclusion

Despite their many cultural differences, families and health professionals do have many goals and aspirations in common. They want to do the "right thing" for the patient, although they may differ on what this entails. They care for and about the patient, although they have different ways of expressing it. Building on the commonalities as well as recognizing the differences are challenges for the future. We must move from culture shock, which many families experience as they encounter the health care system when a relative is seriously ill, to culture change, which involves adapting attitudes, practices, and policies. This will require in-depth research, education, and training and public policies that recognize family caregivers as essential to both individual patient care and the functioning of the health care system.

REFERENCES

Chen, F. M., L. A. Rhodes, and L. A. Green. (2001). "Family Physicians Personal Experiences of Their Fathers' Health Care." *Journal of Family Practice* 50(9):762–66.
Harrington, M. (2000). *Care and Equality.* New York: Routledge.
Kinney, J. M., and M. P. Stephens. (1989). "Caregiving Hassles Scale: Assessing the Daily Hassles of Caring for a Family Member with Dementia." *Gerontologist* 29(3):328–32.
Levine, C., A. Kuerbis, D. A. Gould, M. Navaie-Waliser, P. H. Feldman, and K. A. Donelan. (2000). *Survey of Family Caregivers in New York City: Findings and Implications for the Health Care System.* New York: United Hospital Fund.
Levine, C., and C. Zuckerman. (1999). "The Trouble with Families: Toward an Ethic of Accommodation." *Annals of Internal Medicine* 130:148–52.
Young, C. (2000). First My Mother, Then My Aunt. In *Always On Call: When Illness Turns Families into Caregivers,* ed. C. Levine, 28. New York: United Hospital Fund.

Part I / Perspectives on Family Caregiving

Data, Diversity, and Personal Experience

CHAPTER ONE

Family Caregivers and the Health Care System

Findings from a National Survey

David A. Gould

The different cultures of the formal, professional health care system and the family are brought into persistent, and yet not well understood, connection in the realm of family caregiving. While this volume describes moments of high drama as families try to work with health care professionals and negotiate complex institutions, the largely invisible activities of family caregivers constitute one of the most socially pervasive and enduring interactions of families with the formal care system. And, as many studies have shown, the formal care system could not be sustained without the enormous contributions of family caregivers. So, a better understanding of the nature of the family caregiving—and how it is challenged and shaped by the formal care system—is of vital importance to health care in the United States.

Because so much of what family caregivers do is performed outside of health care institutions or physicians' offices, it is not consistently or accurately measured—an essential first step to insightful analysis. A recent study, however, provides an important measure of the significance of family caregiving to the larger health care system. Arno, Levine, and Memmot (2000) used data from different national population-based surveys to estimate the economic value of informal caregiving in the United States in 1997. They estimated that the value of this caregiving in 1998 was $196 billion—more than the cost of formal home care and nursing home care combined and almost the equivalent of 20 percent of total health care expenditures. Updated projections for 2000 indicate the value has grown to $257 billion (Arno 2002). These are conservative estimates. The authors used mid-range values for numbers of caregivers and wage rates while using only one value for the number of hours of care provided, because only one survey provided national data on the question.

This study also captured the definitional and measurement difficulties that have emerged in research on family caregivers over the past several decades. Studies of so-called informal, or unpaid, caregivers of sick and elderly people proliferated in the 1970s and 1980s. Stimulated by the establishment of Medicare and Medicaid and the expenditure of public funds on medical care, many of these studies focused on program recipients and their caregivers. Other efforts looked at seriously ill people with specific diseases, especially Alzheimer's, to characterize the stress and burden on their caregivers. Although the vast literature has given us much valuable information, most of it was compiled in an era when health care services (and costs) were increasing rapidly, government programs were expanding, and the impact of sophisticated home care technology had yet to be felt. Managed care was still a gleam in a few cost-conscious budgeteers' eyes.

Informal caregivers provide most of the long-term care to elderly or disabled persons living in the community. On this point all sources agree, whether they place the extent of it at 80, 85, or 90 percent. But there is less consensus on the best steps for documenting the vast amount of family care. Questions about how many caregivers there are, what qualifies as caregiving, how much time caregivers spend, and what exactly they do can be answered through several different methodologies. Results that appear inconsistent may actually reflect researchers' varying assumptions and choices.

One problem is that sources count different care recipient and caregiving populations at different times and with different purposes. Some ask care recipients who provides care; others ask caregivers about what they do (usually in terms of assisting care recipients with specific items on a list of Activities of Daily Living [ADLs] or Instrumental Activities of Daily Living [IADLs]) or how burdened they feel by caregiving. Some studies look at specific populations of caregivers, such as those caring for a person with cancer or dementia; others look at caregiving in the broadest sense. Some define *family* narrowly in legal and even tax code terms; others use a broader, more inclusive definition reflecting underlying social realities.

Furthermore, surveys use somewhat different definitions of caregiving. Most surveys use some measure of ADLs, including bathing, toileting, and other forms of personal care; and IADLs, including transportation, shopping, housework, and other types of nonpersonal care. While these are useful to determine the care recipient's functional capacities, they do not reflect the degrees of difficulty inherent in caring for people with various conditions. They do not take into account recent additions to home care of high-tech medical procedures and monitoring. Nor do they document the effort and time involved in patient advocacy, as caregivers negotiate with clinicians, suppliers, health insurance plans, government agencies, and the like in a more bureaucratized, contentious environment. Finally, task-oriented survey questions fail to capture the amount of time caregivers spend just "being there," unable to leave the care recipient alone but not performing a specific task at the moment.

To gain a richer understanding of caregiving, the United Hospital Fund collaborated with several organizations to conduct a national, population-based survey of family caregivers. The national survey, "Long-Term Care from the Caregiver's Perspective," was collaboratively conducted by the Henry J. Kaiser Family Foundation, the Harvard School of Public Health, and the National Opinion Research Center (NORC) at the University of Chicago (Donelan et al. 2002). The United Hospital Fund and the Visiting Nurse Service of New York assisted in developing the survey instrument and interpreting its findings. Funded by the Henry J. Kaiser Foundation, the national survey also included an over-sample of New York City respondents, funded by the United Hospital Fund and the Visiting Nurse Service of New York, to permit an analysis of the city's as well as the nation's experiences.

The survey elicited information about several important but little-studied issues, especially probing the caregivers' relationship with the formal medical care system. Guided by research conducted by the fund (Levine 2000; 2002), the survey attempted to learn more about the transition from hospital to home-based care. Alert to the fact that the discharge process was too often hurried and incomplete, the survey asked family caregivers what sources (if any) of training they had received to prepare them to perform complex medical tasks as well as to assist with ADLs. It also asked who had provided the training. Understanding that rapid transitions do not define the full caregiving experience, which for many family members is a long-term commitment, caregivers were also asked about their interactions over time with staff of the formal health care system, including home care nurses and home health aides. The survey also tried to explore caregiver perceptions of needs that were not met by the formal care system and their understanding of why these needs remained unmet.

This chapter examines some of the findings of the national survey, which portray a compelling picture of caregivers, the people they care for, the variety and intensity of the tasks they perform, their interaction with the formal care system, and their unmet needs for caregiving assistance. (For a more in-depth report of the findings from the New York City survey, see Levine et al. 2000.) This chapter does not discuss data from the New York City survey. Yet its caregivers are quite similar to their counterparts elsewhere in the country, despite major differences in their race, ethnicity, and religion and in the local health care system. This in itself is a major finding, since New York City's health care system, and New Yorkers in general, are often presumed to be very different from the rest of the United States. The experience of family caregiving appears to be a powerfully shared experience across the diversity of the nation.

Survey Design and Sampling

The survey's definition of *caregiver* was deliberately broad:

> Anybody who provides unpaid or arranges for paid or unpaid help to a relative or friend because they have an illness or disability that leaves them unable to do some things for themselves or because they are getting older. This kind of help could be with household chores or finances or with personal or medical needs. The person who needs help may live with you in your home, in their own home, or in another place such as a nursing home.

This definition covers a wide range of relationships and tasks, both those traditionally associated with caregiving as well as activities such as arranging or paying for care. Of the 4,874 respondents who completed the screening interview in early 1998, 1,002 caregivers were identified. (The sample was weighted to reflect the general population, which affects the sample size throughout the report.) Roughly one in five persons (21.8 percent) reported that they were current caregivers or people who had cared for someone within the last twelve months.*

Descriptive Findings

Who Are the Caregivers?

Caregiving is usually assumed to be, and in many respects remains, a woman's role. Nevertheless, this population-based survey identified many more male caregivers than had previous surveys of specific groups of caregivers. Typically, women outnumber men by three to one (NAC/AARP 1997). We found, however, that 53.7 percent of caregivers were female, and 46.3 percent were male (Table 1).

Men and women's roles and assessments of caregiving were different. Men did not provide as much care, as measured in hours per week (as described in Table 1) and in terms of the study's measure of intensity, which will be presented later in this chapter.

Nearly two-thirds (65.3 percent) of the male caregivers provided episodic care or spent nineteen or fewer hours per week; almost a quarter (24.2 percent) provided twenty to fifty-nine hours of care per week; and only 10.5 percent spent sixty or more hours or provided constant care. While more than half of the women (54.9 percent) also provided episodic care or spent nineteen or fewer hours per week, the remainder was evenly divided between those providing twenty to fifty-nine hours; 19 percent provided sixty or more hours per week or constant care (22.4 percent and 22.6 percent, respectively).

Caregivers were also younger than expected (see Table 1). Almost equal proportions were between the ages of eighteen and thirty-nine years and forty and sixty-four years (42.7 percent and 43.9 percent, respectively). Only 13.4 percent were age sixty-five years or older. The projected impact of an aging population on the "baby boomers" is not just a future phenomenon; it has already begun as the boomer generation cares for its parents and grandparents.

More than half of caregivers were employed full-time (52.6 percent), which

*Proportions and percentages may vary slightly from other published works on this data for various reasons, including alternative methods of coding, distinct definitions of variable categorization, use of missing data, and different methods of data cleaning. Despite these minor irregularities, the findings are consistent. In addition, cases were weighted to reflect the general population. As a result, the sample size varies. For a more detailed description of methodologies, refer to Levine et al., 2000.

Table 1. Characteristics of Caregivers

Characteristic	Percentage
Gender (N = 1,063)	
Male	46.3
Female	53.7
Age (N = 1,063)	
18–39	42.7
40–64	43.9
65+	13.4
Employment status (N = 1,059)	
Employed full-time	52.6
Employed part-time	10.6
Not employed	36.8
Marital status (N = 1,059)	
Married	60.0
Not married	40.0
Health status (N = 1,062)	
Excellent	27.7
Very good	29.9
Good	26.2
Fair	13.1
Poor	3.2
Has serious health problem (N = 1,062)	32.3
Primary caregiver (N = 971)	51.1
Current caregiver (N = 1,063)	71.5
Reason for caregiving	
Caregiver lives closest (N = 1,063)	58.2
Caregiver had most time (N = 1,062)	43.2
Recipient wants no strangers in home (N = 1,048)	37.1
No professional help needed (N = 1,054)	43.8
Recipient cannot afford help (N = 1,057)	39.8
Early hospital discharge (N = 1,058)	12.2
Hours of caregiving (N = 1,023)	
1–19, episodic	59.7
20–59	23.3
60+	17.0
Duration of caregiving in years (N = 1,058)	
<1	21.9
1–4	37.3
5+	40.8

is not surprising given their relatively young age. A small percentage had part-time jobs (10.6 percent); the rest were not employed. More than half of the sample (60 percent) were married.

Who Do They Care For?

Most care recipients were female (65.3 percent). Almost two-thirds were older than sixty-four, with 34.7 percent between the ages of sixty-five and seventy-nine years and 30.6 percent age eighty years or older (Table 2). Care recipients between the ages of nineteen and sixty-four years made up 28 percent of the total, and chronically ill or disabled children under eighteen ac-

Table 2. Characteristics of Care Recipients

Characteristic	Percentage
Gender (N = 1,063)	
Male	34.7
Female	65.3
Age (N = 1,030)	
<18	6.7
19–64	28
65–79	34.7
80–89	24.1
90+	6.5
Relationship (N = 1,063)	
Parent	41.8
Other relative	17.5
Grandparent	16.2
Spouse	6.8
Child	5.6
Companion/partner	1.0
Nonrelative/friend	11.1
Residence (N = 1,057)	
Lives alone	37.0
Lives with caregiver	28.8
Lives with family/friend	21.8
Lives in nursing home	7.8
Lives in other group situation	4.6
Other	0
Health status (N = 1,062)	
Excellent	6.0
Very good	15.9
Good	22.5
Fair	29.3
Poor	26.3
Has serious health problem (N = 978)	73.9
Hospitalized in past 12 months (N = 1,060)	54.6

counted for 6.7 percent. It is important to remember that young and middle-aged adults constitute a large portion of persons receiving care.

Care recipients were most often (41.8 percent) the parent of the caregiver. Grandparents constituted 16.2 percent of the care recipients. Other relatives, including aunts, uncles, cousins, siblings, and other family members, accounted for 17.5 percent of care recipients. Another 11.1 percent were non-relatives or friends. Only 6.8 percent of care recipients were spouses, and 1 percent were companions or partners (see Table 2). The relatively small proportion of spouses is likely due to the inclusive criteria for defining caregiving and caregivers as well as the predominance of elderly female care recipients who had never married or had outlived their husbands. More than a third of the care recipients (37 percent) lived alone. Caregivers and care recipients shared a residence in 28.8 percent of the cases, and another 21.8 percent lived in the home of another family member or friend. Only 7.8 percent lived in nursing homes, and 4.6 percent lived in another group living situation.

Caregiver Perspectives

The survey participants reported that the people they care or cared for have serious health problems (see Table 2). Nearly 30 percent of the survey respondents reported that their care recipient was in fair health, while 26.3 percent reported the recipient was in poor health. An even higher percentage of survey respondents (73.9 percent) said the care recipient had a serious health problem. Significantly, 54.6 percent of the care recipients had been hospitalized in the past year.

Caregivers described a range of familiar but serious health problems suffered by care recipients: heart disease, osteoarthritis, diabetes, cancer, and a range of other ailments. Many care recipients had more than one disease. Cognitive impairments—Alzheimer's, senility, and dementia—were reported for roughly one in ten care recipients. These diseases mirror the epidemiology of disease among older people in the United States.

Many caregivers could give only a vague description of the care recipients' health problems or attributed the health problems to "old age." This finding suggests that some health care professionals are not communicating adequately with caregivers about the patient's diagnosis and, by inference, about prognosis and treatment. Also, many caregivers described their loved one's condition as a slow deterioration, caused by one disease, leading to an increased number of ailments, thus making one clear diagnosis difficult.

Caregiver Self-Perceptions

More than half of the caregivers (51.1 percent) reported that they were the primary caregiver; that is, the one who, aside from paid help, "provides/provided most of the care" (see Table 1). A distinction was made between current and not-current caregivers, with *not-current caregivers* defined as those who were not caring for someone at the time of the interview but who had cared for someone at some time in the past twelve months preceding the interview (Levine et al. 2000). In most cases the people for whom they had cared had died, while others recovered or moved to another setting. Not-current caregivers constituted 28.5 percent of the respondents.

When the caregivers were asked why they took on caregiving responsibilities, their reasons varied from the pragmatic to the more subjective (see Table 1). More than half of the caregivers (58.2 percent) reported that they took on this role because they lived closest to the care recipient, and another 43.2 percent reported caregiving because they were the family member with the most time. In contrast to perceptions of comparative convenience, caregivers also reported obstacles to alternative caregiving scenarios. More than a third (37.1 percent) reported that the care recipient did not want strangers in the home. A similar proportion (39.8 percent) of all caregivers said that the care recipient could not afford paid help. A large portion of caregivers (43.8 percent) reported that the care recipient's needs did not require professional help. It was not clear, however, who judged the need for professional help—someone in the formal system, the caregiver, or the care recipient. Only one in eight (12.2 percent) said that the care recipient had been discharged from the hospital too soon.

Finally, it is important to note that caregivers, as a group, are also in vulnerable health. One-third (32.3 percent) report serious health problems of their own (see Table 1).

Caregiving as a Job

Some caregivers spent a lot of time fulfilling their responsibilities; for others the tasks were less time-consuming. Caregivers were asked to estimate the total number of hours per week they spent performing various caregiving tasks or to characterize the time spent as either "episodic" or "constant." Constant care was interpreted to equal sixty hours per week of care and episodic to be only one hour per week of care. By these measures caregivers spent an estimated average of 20.9 hours per week providing care, which is higher than the 1997 National Alliance for Caregiving (NAC) AARP estimate of an average of 17.9 hours per week. Six in ten caregivers (59.7 percent) reported spending less than twenty hours a week or providing episodic care, 23.3 percent reported spending twenty to fifty-nine hours a week, and 17 percent reported spending sixty or more hours per week or providing constant care (see Table 2).

Caregiving for most caregivers lasted a long time (see Table 2). Four in ten caregivers (40.8 percent) reported that they had been caregivers for five or more years. More than a third (37.3 percent) had been caring for one to four years, and only 21.9 percent had been caregivers for less than a year.

Caregivers were asked about specific tasks involved with caregiving, ranging from ADLs and IADLs to medically related tasks (see Table 1). Among the ADLs, which involve personal care, over 25 percent of caregivers performed each task except managing incontinence and feeding, which were performed by 17.2 percent and 16.7 percent of respondents, respectively. More than half the caregivers provided assistance with IADLs, which have more to do with the household and the outside world, except arranging for government assistance through programs such as Medicare or Medicaid. The highest proportion of caregivers performed shopping or errands (84.8 percent); provided transportation, either by driving or by helping with public transportation (75.6 percent); and did housework (71.1 percent).

Given its sharper focus on the possibility of new challenges confronting family caregivers, it is important to note the survey's finding of significant involvement in medically related tasks (Table 3). More than a third of all caregivers (39.1 percent) provided help with prescription medications that were given orally, by injection, intravenously, by infusion pump, or by suppository. Almost a fifth (19.1 percent) changed dressings or bandages, and 14.7 percent helped with medical equipment such as oxygen, home dialysis, tubes, or catheters. Many caregivers are doing far more than personal care and household tasks.

A Measure of Caregiving Intensity

The NAC/AARP study included a Level of Care Index to measure the intensity of caregiving, on a scale of one to five, in which one was the least intensive and five was the most intensive (Levine et al. 2000, 10).Using this measure, we find a rough bell-shaped distribution. Roughly 40 percent of all

Table 3. Tasks Performed by Caregivers

Task	Total Percentage	Care Recipient	
		Hospitalized in Past Year (%)	Not Hospitalized in Past Year (%)
ADLs (N = 981)		(N = 526)	(N = 450)
Bathing	25.6	33.0	20.0
Dressing	41.7	49.3	32.9
Feeding	16.7	21.0	11.8
Incontinence care	17.2	21.1	12.7
Transfer from bed to chair	40.4	52.4	28.0
Walking	34.4	44.3	23.0
IADLs (N = 1,063)		(N = 578)	(N = 481)
Shopping	84.8	89.3	79.0
Housework	71.1	73.0	68.6
Meals	59.2	63.5	53.9
Transportation	75.6	79.2	71.3
Telephone	59.2	64.9	52.2
Finances	48.2	49.5	46.5
Government assistance	29.5	29.9	28.8
Medical			
Dressings (N = 971)	19.1	24.4 (N = 524)	12.9 (N = 443)
Equipment (N = 971)	14.7	20.6 (N = 525)	7.0 (N = 444)
Medications (N = 799)	39.1	43.3 (N = 485)	32.3 (N = 310)
Intensity (N = 977)		(N = 524)	(N = 450)
Level 1	25.1	18.9	31.8
Level 2	14.2	10.3	18.9
Level 3	21.3	24.2	18.0
Level 4	23.5	28.1	18.4
Level 5	15.9	18.5	12.9

Abbreviations: ADL = activities of daily living; IADLs = instrumental activities of daily living

caregivers provided the two lowest levels of care, and a similar proportion provided the two highest levels of care (see Table 3). The experience of caregiving clearly is not driven by large numbers of persons providing small amounts of service, nor are all caregivers consumed by their tasks.

The Impact of Hospitalization

As anticipated, the survey found that hospitalization had a major impact on the type, extent, and duration of care. And it is critically important to remember that 54.6 percent of care recipients had been hospitalized within the past year. In every category of ADL, caregivers were required to do more for care recipients who had been hospitalized in the past year than for those who had not (see Table 3). For example, caregivers looking after someone who had been hospitalized were more than half again as likely to bathe* or manage incontinence† of the care recipient and more than twice as likely to help with dressing,‡ feeding,§ getting in and out of bed,‖ and walking across the room.#

Hospitalization of the care recipient also had an impact on the types of IADLs a caregiver performed, though not as significantly as it did on ADLs (see Table 3). Those caring for a loved one who had been hospitalized were twice as likely to do the shopping** and one and a half times as likely to make telephone calls on behalf of a care recipient†† than caregivers serving persons who had not been hospitalized in the past year. Since most caregivers performed a substantial number of IADLs, regardless of the health status of the care recipient, hospitalization had less relative influence on this measure.

The pattern toward more caregiving following hospitalization was true for medically related tasks as well (see Table 3). Of those caring for persons who had been hospitalized, 24.4 percent changed dressings or bandages, compared to only 12.9 percent of caregivers of persons who had not been hospitalized.‡‡ Also, caregivers providing care for a formerly hospitalized person were almost three times as likely to be helping with medical equipment as those who were caring for someone who had not been hospitalized.§§ Those caring for recently hospitalized persons were only slightly more likely to help with prescription medications as those who were caring for someone who had not been hospitalized,‖‖ which suggests the prevalence of medication use among a largely chronic care population.

Hospitalization had a complex relationship with the intensity and duration of caregiving. While a recent hospitalization did not significantly influ-

*OR = 1.75; 95% CI = (1.3, 2.35); $P < .001$
†OR = 1.8; 95% CI = (1.3, 2.6); $P = .001$
‡OR = 1.9; 95% CI = (1.5, 2.6); $P < .001$
§OR = 2; 95% CI = (1.4, 2.8); $P < .001$
‖OR = 3.02; 95% CI = (2.3, 3.96); $P < .001$
#OR = 2.67; 95% CI = (2.02, 3.52); $P < .001$
**OR = 2.2; 95% CI = (1.56, 3.11); $P < .001$
††OR = 1.7; 95% CI = (1.32, 2.2); $P < .001$
‡‡Hospitalized care recipients, N = 524; nonhospitalized care recipients, N = 443; OR = 2.2; 95% CI = (1.56, 3.08); $P < .001$
§§OR = 2.93; 95% CI = (1.97, 4.38); $P < .001$
‖‖OR = 1.6; 95% CI = (1.2, 2.2); $P = .002$

ence the number of hours of care provided each week, it is interesting to note that those caring for recently hospitalized care recipients were only half as likely to have been longer-term caregivers—more than five years—as compared to those caring for someone who had not been hospitalized within a year.* It is likely that the hospitalization in the past year was the trigger event that precipitated the need for continued caregiving, and the family was the source of that care.

If the duration of care for recently hospitalized persons was shorter, we find dramatic differences between caregiving for a hospitalized and nonhospitalized patient when using the Level of Care Index (see Table 3). Caregivers for the recently hospitalized were twice as likely to be at level 4 or 5 as those caring for a nonhospitalized individual.† Finally, caregivers caring for those hospitalized in the past year were almost twice as likely as someone caring for a nonhospitalized care recipient to hire or arrange for some type of formal home care, such as a nurse or a home care aide.‡

Caregiver Instruction

A disturbing proportion of caregivers reported receiving no instructions for performing caregiving tasks (Table 4). More than half (56.9 percent) of those who performed ADLs reported receiving no instructions for these tasks, some of which require special training and are considerably more difficult and involved when performed for an ill or disabled individual. Almost a third (31.4 percent) of those who changed dressings or bandages, in which technique is clearly important, reported receiving no instruction. Just under a fifth (18.1 percent) of those who helped use medical equipment reported receiving no instruction. A similar proportion (19 percent) of those who administered prescription medications reported that they did not receive instruction for performing the task.

Those who did receive instruction obtained it from either the formal system (nurses, doctors, or their referrals) or informal sources (people whom caregivers identified on their own) (see Table 4). The formal system was most effective in instructing people about medications and using medical equip-

---

*OR = 0.54; 95% CI = (0.43, 0.7); $P < .001$
†OR = 1.9; 95% CI = (1.5, 2.5); $P < .001$
‡OR = 1.9; 95% CI = (1.4, 2.5); $P < .001$

Table 4. Instruction Received by Caregivers

Task	Percentage
ADLs (N = 556)	
No one	56.9
System directed	30.6
Nonsystem	12.5
Not "very comfortable" (N = 562)	34.2
Medications (N = 312)	
No one	19.0
System directed	72.0
Nonsystem	8.9
Not "very capable" (N = 311)	22.1
Bandages (N = 183)	
No one	31.4
System directed	58.7
Nonsystem	9.9
Not "very capable" (N = 185)	30.3
Equipment (N = 142)	
No one	18.1
System directed	69.8
Nonsystem	12.1
Not "very capable" (N = 141)	35.0

ADLs = activities of daily living

ment; nearly three-quarters of caregivers (72 percent and 69.8 percent, respectively) reported receiving some direction from the formal system on these aspects of care. The formal system was not as effective in providing instruction on changing dressings and bandages (58.7 percent). For each medical task some caregivers had to turn to an informal source to find help, which typically was someone they knew, such as a neighbor, a relative with a health care background, or some other acquaintance. Relying on this type of nonsystem instruction injects an element of chance at best and risk at worst.

Full-time employed caregivers were less likely to receive instruction on some medical tasks than other caregivers. For example, caregivers who were employed full-time were less than half as likely to receive system-directed instruction for changing dressings and bandages, as opposed to caregivers who were not employed at the time of the interview.* These caregivers might have been unable to be present when the care recipient was discharged from the hospital or might not have been given other opportunities for instruction.

*OR = 0.39; 95% CI = (0.2, 0.75); $P < .01$

Table 5. *Formal Care Provided Unmet Needs*

Care/Need	Percentage
Paid professional	
None (N = 1,059)	82.3
One or more	17.7
Rated excellent-good (N = 187)	83.0
Rated fair-poor	17.0
Worried (N = 187)	23.3
Aide	
None (N = 1,058)	90.6
One or more	9.4
Rated excellent-good (N = 99)	82.0
Rated fair-poor	18.0
Worried (N = 99)	18.9
Needed help (N = 1,063)	17.9
Medical	55.5
Nonmedical (N = 183)	71.2
Both	26.7
Reason need was unmet (N = 179)	
Access	41.8
Finance	36.4
Family disagreement	21.8

Obtaining Additional Help

Only a small proportion of caregivers (19.9 percent) arranged for or paid for additional formal help, either a professional, such as a nurse or physical therapist, or a paraprofessional, such as a home care aide (Table 5).* Only 17.7 percent of caregivers reported hiring or arranging for one or more paid professionals, and only 9.4 percent of caregivers had hired or arranged for one or more paid home care aides.

Caregivers who hired or arranged for paid help were more than three times as likely as those who had not hired or arranged for paid help to be at levels 4 and 5 of the Level of Care Index.† Clearly, paid assistance did not release caregivers from their roles but, rather, supplemented their very considerable level of service. Significant needs following a hospitalization may be the key factor contributing to this pattern.

*N = 1,057. The wording of the question allows for the possibility that more people received formal care than the question captured. This finding is consistent, however, with other national studies, in which the vast majority of people receive only "informal" care.

†OR = 3.6; 95% CI = (2.6, 5); $P < .001$

The caregivers' perceptions of this additional formal assistance are mixed. The overwhelming majority of caregivers who had hired or arranged for paid help in the past year reported good to excellent quality of care by both paid professionals (83 percent) and home care aides (82 percent) (see Table 5). Nevertheless, a notable proportion of the small number of caregivers who hired or arranged for paid help reported worrying about mistreatment or neglect of their care recipient by both professionals (23 percent) and paraprofessionals (19 percent).

Unmet Needs for Caregiving Assistance

Caregivers were asked whether they had needed but could not get help caring for the care recipient in the past year. If they answered yes, they were asked if their needs were medical, nonmedical, or both (see Table 5). Almost a fifth of the sample (17.9 percent) reported that they needed but could not get help within the past year. More than half of those caregivers (55.5 percent) reported unmet medical needs, such as a nurse for the care recipient, and 71.2 percent reported an unmet nonmedical need for assistance, such as a home care aide.

Caregivers gave their own answers about the reasons for unmet needs, which were grouped into the following categories:

- access-related difficulties, which included refusal of service by doctors or hospitals, problems with services or transportation, the lack of an available doctor or nurse, or a "government decision" that the care recipient did not need the services (41.8 percent);
- financial difficulties, which included the inability to pay for services, insurance problems, and ineligibility for government assistance based on income or financial assets (36.4 percent); and
- family problems, which included disagreements within the family about who should provide care, not having enough time or strength, or caregiver illness (21.8 percent).

Clearly, caregivers who report unmet needs perceive that the obstacles to care in the main reflect some type of systemic problem and are not the result of familial disagreements or the inability of the family to marshal its own caregiving resources.

Perspectives on Caregiver Competence

Caregivers were also surveyed on their perceived levels of comfort and capability in providing care. Those who reported that they performed ADLs, or medical tasks, were asked how comfortable or capable they felt about performing these tasks (see Table 5). A third (34.2 percent) of those performing ADLs felt "not at all comfortable," "not very comfortable," or "somewhat comfortable." Two-thirds reported being "very comfortable" performing ADLs.

When asked how capable they felt about performing medical tasks such as changing dressings or bandages or helping with medical equipment, close to a third of the respondents (30.3 percent) did not feel totally capable of managing dressings and bandages or with helping with medical equipment (35.0 percent). When asked about managing prescription medications, however, a smaller but still high percentage (22.1 percent) said they felt less than completely capable.

But caregivers responded even more negatively when asked about the overall experience of caregiving than when asked about specific tasks. In evaluating caregiving as an overall experience, 33.8 percent reported that it was "somewhat difficult," and 8.7 percent said it was "very difficult" (a total of 42.5 percent). Only 34.6 percent reported that it was "not at all difficult," and 22.9 percent said it was not "very difficult."

Those who spent twenty hours or more a week caregiving were twice as likely as those who devoted fewer than twenty hours per week to report that it was somewhat or very difficult.* This finding is particularly instructive. Surveys that look only at tasks performed to measure burden may miss this dimension: caregivers assess difficulty not just by tasks but by the whole experience. And persons providing more care do not necessarily develop a greater sense of competence and self-assurance.

Implications for the Health Care System

This survey demonstrates the spectrum of caregiving experiences and the heterogeneity of caregivers. Caregivers provide a significant amount of care to

*OR = 1.8; 95% CI = (1.4, 2.3); $P < .001$

their ill, disabled, and elderly relatives and friends. For the most part they provide even intense care with little or no paid help. This survey also documents the extent to which hospitalization is a key transition point for caregivers. This finding supports the qualitative data reported in Levine (1998) and the strategy of the United Hospital Fund's Family Caregiving Grant Initiative, which has awarded two million dollars to seven New York City hospitals to develop educational and support programs for caregivers and professional staff.

The survey findings also highlight the need to better define and measure caregiver activities in order to capture the full range and complexity of caregiver tasks beyond the commonly used ADL-IADL measures. Such measures should take into account current medical home care technologies and difficult personal care. They should also include the often underestimated tasks of care management, navigation of the health care and social services systems, and patient care advocacy. Ideally, the measures should reflect the variability in difficulty depending on the patient's condition, the home environment, and the family's caregiving capacity. Without such measures it will be difficult to document the multiple roles that caregivers play or the areas in which additional training and support will yield the greatest benefits for caregivers, care recipients, and health care workers. (The United Hospital Fund is working with grant support from the Robert Wood Johnson Foundation to examine the shortfalls of currently used measures and to identify promising approaches.)

The survey pointedly documents that many caregivers are not receiving instruction to prepare them for the increased responsibilities that follow hospitalization. It is clear that hospital discharge planners are not helping all caregivers put in place appropriate home health services in the post–acute care period. Hospitals must do a better job of training and educating caregivers and must work with community-based agencies to follow up with additional services, training, and monitoring as needed. In this regard it is also important to develop and test more effective ways to train caregivers both to perform specific tasks and to relieve their overall difficulty. In this area it is critical to understand the dynamics of interpersonal relationships involving caregivers, professionals, paraprofessionals, and care recipients. Studies should explore the impact of caregiver training and support on care recipients' recovery or stabilization and the subsequent use of medical services, including readmission to hospitals.

Although this survey could not measure the quality of care provided by family caregivers, it seems apparent that people who have not been trained cannot recognize or report such lapses in quality. Some of these lapses are not serious, while others may result in rehospitalization or the patient's deteriorated condition. At the same time, family caregivers cannot be held to institutional standards of care that are possible in a hospital with shifts of staff and other resources.

Insurance companies, government payers, and managed care companies must recognize that it is essential to train and support caregivers and reimburse providers adequately for these services. A single-minded focus on reducing costs ignores the health impact on the caregiver, with resulting poorer health status for the caregiver as well as impaired quality of care for the care recipient.

The survey demonstrates that for many caregivers the formal health care system is difficult to understand and access—and for some it is quite threatening. It is important to help caregivers manage and navigate the health care system; identify and address the factors contributing to distrust of the home care workforce; and explore ways to mitigate the impact of long-term and heavy-duty caregiving. In particular, home care organizations must address the widespread distrust about the home care workforce. This distrust may be influenced by media reports of fraud and abuse. It was expressed in the survey data by caregivers who either had hired or arranged for paid help or who did not have paid help because of concern about having a stranger in the home. Caregivers' concerns must be addressed candidly and forthrightly so that those who need help can confidently welcome workers into their homes or the homes of their loved ones.

Conclusion

In summary, caregiving across the nation is pervasive and private. Roughly one in five adults provides some level of caregiving; nearly 85 percent had not hired or arranged for paid home health aides or professionals in the past year.

Hospitalization of the care recipient is a key event for caregivers. Increased levels of care and responsibilities are likely to follow. Hospitals have a responsibility to patients and caregivers to ensure continuity and quality of care and adequate support for caregivers.

Caregivers are not receiving adequate training to prepare them for their responsibilities. Hospitals, providers, and home care agencies have a responsibility to ensure that caregivers obtain proper instruction about techniques of caregiving, preventing medication errors, maintaining infection control, and other aspects of caregiving. Support for the emotional aspects of caregiving is an essential part of this training.

Insurance companies, government payers, and managed care companies should recognize that training and support of caregivers is an essential aspect of patient care and should adequately reimburse providers for this service.

Formal caregivers, especially home care agencies, should examine the reasons for the widespread worry about mistreatment or neglect of care recipients and should correct any systemic problems to build trust among caregivers.

REFERENCES

Arno, P. S. "Economic Value of Informal Caregiving." (2002, Feb. 22). Paper presented at the annual meeting of the American Association for Geriatric Psychiatry, Orlando, Fla.

Arno, P. S., C. Levine, and M. M. Memmot. (1999). "The Economic Value of Informal Caregiving." *Health Affairs* 18(2):182–88.

Donelan, K., C. A. Hill, C. Hoffman, K. Scoles, P. H. Feldman, C. Levine, and D. A. Gould. (2002). "Challenged to Care: Informal Caregivers in a Changing Health System." *Health Affairs* 21(4):222–31.

Emanuel, E. J., D. L. Fairclough, J. Slutsman, H. Alpert, D. Baldwin, and L. L. Emanuel. (1999). "Assistance from Family Members, Friends, Paid Caregivers, and Volunteers in the Care of Terminally Ill Patients." *New England Journal of Medicine* 341(13):956–63.

Emanuel, E. J., D. L. Fairclough, J. Slutsman, and L. L. Emanuel. (2000). "Understanding Economic and Other Burdens of Terminal Illness: The Experience of Patients and Their Caregivers." *Annals of Internal Medicine* 132:451–59.

Levine, C. (1998). *Rough Crossings: Family Caregivers' Odysseys through the Health Care System.* New York: United Hospital Fund.

Levine, C., A. N. Kuerbis, D. A. Gould, M. Navaie-Waliser, P. H. Feldman, and K. Donelan. (2000). *A Survey of Family Caregivers in New York City: Findings and Implications for the Health Care System.* New York: United Hospital Fund, with the Visiting Nurse Service of New York.

National Alliance for Caregiving (NAC) AARP. (1997). *Family Caregiving in the U.S., Findings from a National Survey.* Washington, D.C.

CHAPTER TWO

On Loving Care and the Persistence of Memories

Reflections of a Grieving Daughter

Gladys Gonzalez-Ramos

I have been fretting about this day, in fact this very hour of this day, for many months. What a relief it will be when midnight finally comes and goes, and I know that I have stared at my inner sadness straight on and have conquered today.

A student of mine gave me a card that says, "In the presence of trouble some people buy crutches, others grow wings." This past year I have been trying to grow wings, to soar mighty and high above the cauldron of feelings threatening to spill over. Yet secretly I know that at any time, at any moment, not having grown mighty wings I might actually need crutches or perhaps a wheelchair to sit on and let someone else carry the weight of my grief, the weight of my loss for my parents, who died together last year, this very day, this very hour.

I can close my eyes and still see it vividly. Early Sunday morning, October 18, 1998, held the promise of a warm, sunny day with the smells of autumn just beginning and the foliage at its peak. I took a long car ride with my friends to buy some things my mother needed and to put some distance from the sadness of having been with my parents two days earlier. Taking my mother on yet another doctor's visit had been so despairing. There was no hope left for her condition, just years waiting to be lived out in slow, chronic deterioration. After the doctor's visit, I had left her at home with her feet dangling up in the air, her body in spasms, and her face showing unspeakable grief. She had lost her life; she had lost her joy; she had lost her smile. The lines on her face, placed there by wrenching sadness and hopelessness, were as raw as my own heart felt upon seeing her like this. As I drove away that Friday after dropping my parents off at their apartment, I suddenly stopped, turned around, and gave my father some Life Savers, which I had in my pocket. I asked him to give them to her; she always liked the cherry-flavored Life Savers. At that moment I felt it was all I had left to offer.

This would be my last act of love and care for my parents. Two days later that beautiful Sunday would not be a day full of promise and hope, as it seemed in the early morning hours; by the end of the day I would be talking to police detectives and medical examiners, making funeral arrangements for both of my parents.

Leaving Home

The day my only brother left Cuba is another day that stays vividly in my memory. December 20, 1960, was a day of partings and a sad day of good-byes. I thought my older brother, barely eleven years old, was the best, brightest, and most handsome person. In my blinding childhood idealization all his faults could be forgiven. I even named my favorite doll after him. And that doll, which I still have today, traveled with me from Cuba.

In the Cuban airport named after José Martí, half of the departure area is enclosed in glass. The *eresa,* as they call it—the fishbowl—serves cruelly to separate the people departing from those staying behind. Loved ones seem so near and yet are so far. I tried to squish my six-year-old body as close as I could to the thick glass wall as my brother stood opposite looking at me. I placed my hands against the glass trying magically to touch his hands, to feel him again. At one point someone opened the door, and through the crack, with a couple of my fingers, I tried to touch him one last time. I wanted to suck him right over to my side of the wall and run all the way home to play our favorite games in our bedroom, to stay next to him forever and never let him go. It would be more than a year and a half before my parents and I would come to New York and be reunited with him. The pain of this separation never fully healed. It is a memory that I am starting to realize has left ripples in all of our lives.

Mine is a Cuban refugee's story, one that resembles in certain ways so many other immigrant stories. The themes set out when I was five years old—when my parents knew that they would have to leave Cuba—have shaped my personal and professional life. The myriad of scars left over from the refugee or immigrant experience often endures and many times goes unnoticed, yet it is these enduring and underlying experiences and the cultural ways of being which shape our entire life cycles, from early child rearing to taking care of our elders.

It was these leftover scars that came to haunt my parents when sickness arrived at their door. My father, who had a major heart attack within months of his retirement, fought this unexpected setback with the resilience, perseverance, and strength he had shown in his years as a Cuban refugee. After undergoing a successful quadruple bypass surgery, he gave up fried food, attended nutrition classes, went to the gym, and took up painting as a hobby. He was the picture of health in his early seventies.

A man full of determination, my father left behind his printing business in Cuba at age forty, not knowing a word of English, and reestablished himself quite successfully in New Jersey. My mother, a woman who knew too much about illness and death from her own family, had been by my father's side since adolescence. They made an incredible team with different yet complementary temperaments. The tune of my father's life was that of a trumpet, full of vigor, energy, promise, and passion; my mother was like a saxophone—steady, smooth, and quiet but consistently strong. His energy and determination would blast out of him. Hers was the steady beat, with the depth required to understand their dreams and help achieve them to their full potential. The two found harmony in each other's melodies during their fifty-two-year marriage.

As my parents' caskets lay beside each other in the funeral home, many of their friends commented on how right it was for them to die as they had lived, side by side.

Seeking Care

My mother's Parkinson disease, diagnosed as my father recovered from his heart attack, was not met with the same sense of hope as my father's heart problem. For him there was an almost perfect cure; there was hope of a good recovery. For her there was a life of slow and chronic deterioration until eventually, ten years after the initial diagnosis, her muscles would go one by one and she could no longer walk, feed, dress, or bathe herself. Cruelly, as her body gave out, enough of her mind was left that she was aware of her deterioration and the dyskinesias that made her twist and shake for hours. She called herself *un payaso,* a clown, a futile attempt at humor to make herself and others more comfortable with the alien spasms that had become her body. My father would tell me in our numerous phone conversations that he slowly had come to accept her physical deterioration, but he could not bear her fading away. The disease was extinguishing her personality and her essence. He would say, "Se esta apagando": she is fading out just like a candle slowly dies.

Culture shapes a family's life from the small daily habits to annual holiday rituals, from the passing of birthdays to funerals. My parents embraced the United States and were forever thankful to have found a new home full of freedom and the ability to educate their children under democratic principles. Yet, when my mother's illness came, they felt the great absence of their own language, their extended families, and a health care system that could respond to their cultural framework and speak their language.

It proved impossible to get comprehensive care for my mother, who not only had complicated and unpredictable physical symptoms but also suffered from the loss of her independence, the loss of her sense of privacy, indeed the loss of life as she had lived it. In the ten years she lived with Parkinson's we would seek help from many excellent neurologists and other specialists. They helped in limited ways, trying to control her bodily symptoms and later on the multiple and cruel side effects of the medications. The doctors inquired extensively about my mother's neurological symptoms. My father had to keep intricate charts on an hourly basis for months trying to pin down her many symptoms and the wild fluctuations brought about by the very medications that were supposed to help her. But it was all fragmented care. For all those years, during which I usually went to the medical appointments with them, no one asked about her emotional well-being, no one considered the permanent sadness and hopelessness that overtook my father's expressions. No one asked about the many psychological needs my parents had in facing a complicated illness like Parkinson's.

Perhaps it was the physicians' own sense of helplessness and hopelessness that made them increasingly reductionistic about my mother's condition. They seemed to see only a partial picture, so they only gave partial help. These were caring professionals with good intentions. But they seemed unable to look beyond my mother's neurological problems and respond to her as a whole person, a person whose essence was fading in front of all of us. They seemed unable to respond to my father's sadness. Perhaps they did notice and just didn't know what to say, but not to inquire, simply to ignore it, was far worse. They might have underestimated the power of what they could do: they could ask, they could listen, they could refer us to other services, they could raise questions to think about—did we need respite care, a wheelchair, a hospital bed, a nursing home? Despite seeking care for my mother from the top medical centers in New York City, I never found the team approach necessary for responding to the multiple, complex, and changing needs of a complicated health problem like Parkinson's. Instead, everything was left to me, their daughter and a social worker. I often wondered what immigrants do who don't have a bilingual social worker as a daughter.

In talks with my father over the last years, Cuba found a way back into our conversations. In the face of the great loss of his life partner, other losses came back to haunt him. He longed for Cuba—not the real Cuba of today but the Cuba of his dreams, the one frozen in his memory. In this Cuba he could speak the right language, had the right accent, and would not have needed to rely on me to negotiate their health care. In the Cuba of his dreams he would have had plenty of family around to offer emotional support. The family would not have been scattered over New York, New Jersey, Florida, and Cuba. The family would have given birth to children who spoke Spanish, and my father would not feel like an outsider with younger members of the family, who were more comfortable with English. He would not feel the humiliation of lacking fluency in English in front of doctors and other authority figures. His daughter would not have had to translate pamphlets given to him at the hospital to explain the sexual dysfunctions that might be side effects of his surgeries. Sometimes I also wished for this Cuba. Now that I am comfortable enough in the United States, I have the luxury of longing and thinking of Cuba. When the Cuban psychologist Olivia Espín returned to Cuba over twenty years after she left, she wrote that "it takes an experience like going back to Cuba to realize that what you have mistaken for comfort does not compare with what the feeling of belonging really means" (1997, 155). But the Cuba my father spoke of existed only in his dreams, in the life he imagined he would have had if he had been able to raise us in a free Cuba. It was a Cuba frozen in time.

Many immigrants hold a frozen, idealized image of their homeland as it might have been when they departed for political or economic reasons. Often the loss of the homeland cannot be fully grieved for many years, if ever. Survival and the need to "make it" take priority. Yet at times of stress, illness, and probably death, a sense of loss may be keen. People may long for the old home and its familiar, soothing smells and rhythms even while recognizing that the medical care in the mainland United States is excellent. But for most immigrants there is no going back. In reality home is often not better; whatever led them to leave is still there. The challenge, then, may be to make the services here more like those of home, more congruent with their culture and language.

The Values of Home

It can be difficult to decipher the essence of my family's cultural values. Except for my father, those in my family have lived longer in this country than we lived in Cuba, and our lifestyles and values reflect in many ways not only Cuban values but also those we have absorbed from the United States. Yet the process of acculturation does not wipe out an essential core of one's culture. My family members and me carry parts of Cuba in us. We carry its idealized image, its language, its food, and its music. The Cuban mental health professionals G. Bernal and E. Shapiro stated, "The story of the Cuban-American family experience must be told as an intergenerational narrative of love, loyalty, and longing" (1996, 155–68). Love and loyalty for the family and longing for the lost home—these core values are found in Cubans today in Miami and West New York, New Jersey. Like other Latino groups in the United States, Cubans tend to work with a collectivistic view of the self as opposed to an individualistic and autonomous self. The family, both blood and nonblood relatives, and loyalty of and to this family are essential to the Cuban sense of self.

Language can often serve as a window to show us what a culture values. In English several expressions reflect the Anglo-American view of the individual as primarily a separate and autonomous person. "Give me space" and "I need some distance" have a special psychological meaning in addition to their concrete sense of needing to be away from others. In contrast, if translated into Spanish, such phrases would be taken only concretely. Language cannot depict a value to which the culture does not adhere. As for the Latin view of the self, what better example can I provide than to say that a spider plant, whose leaves arch out and away from the plant and create new plants where they touch the ground, is known by Cubans and other Latinos as *mala madre,* bad mother? In this worldview a mother should not allow her children to leave the family nest.

By extension, in the Cuban perspective the nest or home is seen as an ever-receptive place for the family. When relatives visit, even for extended periods, one should naturally open one's doors. And, when family members become sick or elderly and can no longer stay in their own home, they naturally expect to move in with their children or other family members. If someone requires hospitalization, the typical expectation is for family members to stay overnight at the hospital. To do otherwise is not to care and not to fulfill one's caregiving responsibilities.

While devotion to the family remains a central value in Cuban values, it is starting to show some wear and tear under the influences of immigration and acculturation. During immigration the nuclear and extended families tend to separate, and many families never reunite physically or psychologically. Indeed, the trends toward urbanization and increased mobility bring about much greater separation. In addition, the housewife's traditional role of staying home to care for the youngsters and the elderly has rapidly changed. These social changes have pushed some Latino families to place the elderly in nursing homes, although this is certainly not a popular solution.

At times social class overrides cultural norms. No matter what the culture is, having money opens doors. Having money allows one to hire live-in help. Having money has allowed a series of Latino homeowners in the Miami area to set up "nursing homes" in their homes to take care of someone else's elderly family members. The family visits as often as they want, bringing their own home-cooked meals, their own linens, and even their own furniture if they wish, while the owners hire the necessary nursing staff to care for the elderly. It is a type of foster group home with cultural values at the center of care. But the poor cannot offer or make use of such options.

Inadequate Alternatives

Years after the initial diagnosis, my mother started to fall more frequently. For a few years she and my father managed as best they could. They prized their independence and their privacy, and she had not wanted any help at home. One of these falls, however, sent her into the hospital, and she was then transferred to a nursing home. She needed rehabilitation, he needed respite, and we needed to see if a home was a viable alternative.

Fearing this decision, I had been researching nursing homes for several months, and I had found myself in a dilemma. The local nursing homes with plenty of Spanish-speaking patients and staff received rather low ratings from the state. Yet the best nursing home, a much newer facility—bright, clean, and attached to the hospital—had almost no Spanish-speaking patients. My parents had lived in this country for over thirty years, but they had never mastered English fluently. Working day and night, they had no time to study the language. They had ended up with Spanish-speaking coworkers, and they established their own business in New Jersey in a Spanish-speaking neighborhood. They had learned enough English to get by but not enough to negotiate a complicated health care system. This was my father's greatest regret and source of humiliation.

We live under the illusion that there are enough Spanish-speaking professionals in such areas as health care because there are so many Latinos in the United States, particularly in places like New York City. This is not the case. All the cardiologists recommended for my father in the New York area spoke only English. My mother saw only one Spanish-speaking neurologist with a specialty in movement disorders in Miami. When my father became my mother's primary caregiver, I could not find a single Spanish-speaking support group for him in either New York City or New Jersey. In fact, when I inquired at various organizations and agencies about such groups, they asked me to volunteer and start one myself. I wished I had the energy to do so, but I often felt that I needed my own support group.

The nursing home we chose was clean and bright, with adequate staff. They made every attempt to make the place cheery, with bright ghosts and goblins at Halloween time and weekly dancing classes, but it proved to be a nightmare. The stench of sadness could not be covered over. My mother, who had tried to carry her illness with her equanimity and faith in God, fell into a

depression. In her early seventies she was one of the youngest patients, surrounded by people with advanced Alzheimer's and other dementias who, if
they spoke at all, spoke only English. My father spent his days by her side, providing companionship and continuing to help her. He had his friends, hob-
bies, and associations he belonged to, but he could not enjoy these while she
lay depressed and alone in the home. He felt lost without her. And she so
wanted to be home.

After several weeks of this, after much crying and looking at various im-
perfect solutions, we took her home. We hired multiple aides because we
needed two at a time in order to care for her and prevent my father from further straining himself. Partly because we needed multiple aides, my parents
were forced to move. Their apartment was too small to house live-in help.
Also, it was a second-floor walk-up, and my mother could no longer negotiate
the stairs. After much thinking, we moved them from their small Spanish-
speaking community in New Jersey to Queens, New York, where we had more
family. This was a great loss for my father, who was tied to his community,
friends, and associations. In fifty years together they had never faced such a
dilemma—what was best for my father was not best for my mother.

I ended up hiring four immigrant aides to care for my mother. While they
spoke Spanish, they could not take her to her medical appointments because
they did not speak English. They were from different South American coun-
tries, and often differing national views and old rivalries would interfere in
their living together. There were different customs, different foods, different
sayings. No matter what arrangements my father and I made, my mother's
longing for privacy with her husband never stopped. They now slept in separate bedrooms, and the evening aide reported that my mother called out for
my father endlessly until the morning hours. Inevitably, my father often
heard my mother calling for him and went to her side, but the stress started
giving him chest pains.

As his own sadness worsened I was able to convince him to go to a
Spanish-speaking psychiatrist—at the very least for symptom relief. The anti-
depressant Zoloft did help his appetite improve and his insomnia decrease.
But here, too, the medical help was partial. The psychiatrist would see my
father only once a month, perhaps for twenty minutes, mainly to write a
prescription. At times, if my father needed to change his appointment, the
psychiatrist might not even return his phone calls. He seemed to see his role

as a psychopharmacologist, not as someone needing to attend to the sadness that Zoloft cannot repair.

He had to talk about his losses to someone other than his daughter. He promised he would go with me to a Cuban social worker I had found so he could talk about what was happening and perhaps start to find other ways to cope. Yet we never made it there. In the early afternoon of October 18, following a well-thought-out plan, he used a gun to kill my mother, and then, positioning himself on the window ledge of their eleventh floor apartment so that he would be knocked out the window by the blast, he shot himself once in the mouth.

It is easy to judge my father from afar, but one is likely to reach the wrong conclusions. My father did not have a history of violence, alcoholism, or depression and had never owned a gun. In the twenty letters he left behind he explains his reasoning. They had lived a long and happy life together. They had traveled and prospered, and they did not want to end their lives in slow deterioration. They wanted to die as they lived, side by side. They wanted to stop the interminable suffering. And it was clear to me that, while he took the action that brought about their death, she had reached the same decision. She would never tell me, but she had been telling the aides in the last few weeks of her life that she wanted to die.

Returning Home

I understood, perhaps too well, my father's last courageous act. It showed the same spirit he had shown as an immigrant when he arrived here in 1961. Yet I wonder if the suffering they went through, especially the last few years, could have been ameliorated. Nothing could have cured my mother's Parkinson's, and, frankly, I don't know if anything could have stopped my father from killing himself and my mother. But I think that we need to find ways to provide health care that is guided by more holistic and humanistic principles. We may be years away from finding the cure for diseases like Parkinson's, but in the meantime there is much that we can do to care for those afflicted with them.

I long for the day when the whole patient and family are placed at the center of care; when a patient is not reduced to mere symptoms and the family caregivers are ignored; when health care is not fragmented; when professional roles are not so rigidly defined; when someone responds both to the diseases of the body and the diseases of the heart and soul. I long for the day when we understand that responding to the multiple needs associated with complicated illnesses requires a team approach.

I also long for the day when the patient's culture is recognized as one of the factors that influence how people express their illnesses and needs and that our ways of helping them must attempt to be congruent with their cultural perspective. I long for the day when patients of limited economic means, which includes the majority of Latinos in the United States, have the options available to those in better economic situations. I long for the day when more health care professionals speak different languages, offer patient forms and pamphlets in other languages, and have capable translators at health care centers. I long for the day when people like my father do not feel that only by killing themselves and their loved ones can they find peace.

An immigrant's longing for the homeland is never laid to rest. It creeps up on us at the most unexpected times, in the most unexpected ways. When the police allowed me to reenter my parent's apartment a week after I had buried them, I found the sheet that covered the chair my mother sat on when my father killed her. It was drenched with her blood, some of the bones from her skull, and a bullet the police had not recovered. By the window ledge I found more bits and pieces of bones from my father's body. I ask you, what does one do with such things? Sweep them up and throw them away with the day's garbage?

I have found the answer after much soul searching. It came from my husband, himself Puerto Rican, who understands so well the longing for one's home. I will—soon, I hope—return to Cuba to bury them back home. My parent's bodies will always remain buried in their beloved community in New Jersey, where they lived and worked, but part of them needs to go back to Cuba.

ACKNOWLEDGMENTS

This chapter is adapted from a presentation to members of The Hastings Center–United Hospital Fund Working Group on the "Cultures of Caregiving," October 18, 1999, which was published in the *Hastings Center Report* 30(4) (2000): 28–33, under the title "The 18th of October 1999: In Memoriam." The material is used here with permission from the Hastings Center.

A detailed account of my parents' story and my role as a family caregiver appears in "The Courage of Caring," in *Always on Call: When Illness Turns Families into Caregivers,* ed Carol Levine, 2d ed. (Nashville: Vanderbilt University Press, 2004).

REFERENCES

Bernal, G., and E. Shapiro. (1996). "Cuban Families." In *Ethnicity and Family Therapy,* ed. M. McGoldrick, J. K. Pearce, and J. Giordano, 2d ed. New York: Guilford Press.
Espin, O. (1997). "Roots Uprooted." In *Latina Realities*. Boulder, Colo.: Westview Press Harper Collins Publishers.

CHAPTER THREE

The Weight of Shared Lives

Truth Telling and Family Caregiving

Jerome K. Lowenstein

When family caregiving is an important component in the treatment of chronic illness, it creates circumstances that challenge many of the accepted paradigms of the patient-physician relationship. Family members in their own or the patient's home now take over responsibility for aspects of care—incontinence care and bathing, administration of medications, monitoring of vital signs, and responding to symptoms—which until recently were in the purview of hospital nurses or other professional personnel. Beyond these roles family caregivers serve as observers, interpreting the physician's words and responses to questions from the patient and others.

When the caregiver is a member of the patient's immediate or even extended family, a unique dynamic is created. The family caregiver and the patient almost always share a history and often a background that are different from those of the physician. Unlike the hospital or in-patient hospice setting, where men or women who are part of the "medical community" provide care, family caregiving occurs in the patient's realm, isolating the physician from the culture of the patient and his or her family caregiver. In one memorable case I found myself as a physician at odds with my patient's family caregiver over the question of truth telling.

The Case of Mr. and Mrs. N

I was totally unprepared when Mr. N's wife said bluntly to me, "You cannot tell him that he has cancer." Mr. N, a Hungarian-born lawyer in his seventies, had been under my care for about ten years. He had mild high blood pressure but had been generally well and was still working at his law practice. He had noticed a fever and a persistent cough that lasted several weeks. A chest X ray revealed a small patch of pneumonia. When he failed to improve with antibiotic treatment, he was hospitalized; a chest CAT scan revealed several lung masses. After some hesitation, he agreed to a transthoracic needle biopsy. He was still in the hospital when I received the pathology report indicating "well differentiated adenocarcinoma"—in other words, metastatic lung cancer.

Mr. N's wife, whom I had met many times during his office visits over the years, was waiting for me outside her husband's hospital room. I explained that the lung biopsy had confirmed my suspicion of a malignancy. She asked what I intended to do, and I explained that further diagnostic tests should be performed. She was attentive but showed little emotional response until she stated, in a manner that made it quite clear that she was well prepared for this moment, that under no circumstances was I to tell her husband the diagnosis. She said that he would not question my ordering further X rays or other tests (looking for a primary lesion) if I explained that they were "necessary for further treatment."

I tried to convince her that it was important for me to maintain an honest relationship with Mr. N. I explained that, although no further treatment was required at this time, my deception would be apparent as his disease progressed and would then make it difficult for me to care for him. She had obviously prepared herself for this argument too and said simply that she would worry about that in the future and would find, perhaps with my help, another physician at such time. I said I would delay for a while my discussion with her husband, and we agreed to talk in my office the following day.

Long discussions with one of my colleagues with a strong background in bioethics did not make the matter much clearer for me. When we met the following day, Mrs. N explained that her husband had always been given to periods of depression; she feared that hearing that he had cancer might "push him over the edge." This judgment was supported by a phone call to Mr. N's daughter and to a physician who had treated him for depression some years earlier. Still, I wondered if Mrs. N was acting in her husband's best interest or in her own. Was she simply denying the terrible fact that he had metastatic cancer and, in a way, forcing me to be an accomplice in that denial?

As we went on, it became clear that, although Mrs. N had always struck me as a bit impatient and critical with her husband, she was in fact intensely devoted to him and was committed to protecting him at any cost. The repercussions when the deception was revealed would surely be worse for her than for me. Yet I found myself struggling to find some way to convince Mrs. N that her husband should be told that he had cancer. I had discussed my patient's management with two oncologists, who felt that, given the clinical information, chemotherapy or radiation therapy had little to offer Mr. N. Reluctantly I agreed to a course of action—withholding the diagnosis—which would have been my first response twenty years earlier but which now left me unsure and uncomfortable. I have often thought back to my decision.

Mr. N accepted the news that he had a "complicated pneumonia" and that, after completing a course of antibiotics, he could leave the hospital to be followed by an appointment in my office. The next year was uneventful for Mr. N; he came to see me for regular visits every two or three months and never again commented about his "pneumonia." About eighteen months later Mrs. N called to report that her husband had been admitted to another hospital, critically ill with anemia and jaundice. He died several days later.

Mrs. N thanked me for the care I had given to her husband. I thought that something in her tone of voice or the words she spoke also expressed her gratitude to me for agreeing to withhold the diagnosis from her husband. I recognize, in retrospect, that Mrs. N was probably correct in her judgment. I came to respect the strong way in which she resisted my arguments, which I had presented in a manner that implied that they reflected the best opinion of the medical community. Was it reasonable for me to decide, unilaterally, that he should be told the truth in order to protect the integrity of my relationship with him?

My long discussions with Mrs. N made it clear that, although Mr. N was my patient and his wife was not, they had shared a long, rich, and at times difficult life together, initially in Hungary and then in New York City. In the end I think it was the realization that I had a responsibility to Mrs. N, as well as to my patient, which governed my decision.

Communicating the "Whole Truth"

It is in the area of communication, and particularly communication related to truth telling, that the differences between the cultures of medicine and the cultures of families may be the most significant. It is well recognized that concepts of illness and strongly held views concerning truth telling vary considerably among individuals, within families, and among cultures. When I first wrote about this case in 1997, my thoughts were focused on what I saw as the conflict between my responsibility to my patient and his wife's demands. There was little question in my mind, after consultation with my oncologist colleagues, that any decisions regarding Mr. N' s medical treatment, defined narrowly as radiation therapy or chemotherapy, would not be influenced by his knowing or not knowing that he had metastatic cancer.

Yet medical treatment goes far beyond the issue of whether the patient is told the diagnosis. The words physicians speak to patients often linger in their minds and in their memories. They are repeated, examined, and reexamined as patients seek reassurance, guidance, or solace. All physicians have heard patients repeat their words or the words of other physicians years after they were spoken. I am quite sure that there are times when what has been said has had greater consequences for the patient's well-being than the medications or treatments prescribed. What is said to a patient or a patient's family should reflect the physician's fullest understanding of all the needs of the patient in the same way as the choice of a medication or advice regarding surgery must consider all the ramifications.

For some patients and family members this will require "full disclosure," by which I mean an effort to fully educate them, recalling that the Latin root of the word *doctor* is *docere,* meaning "to teach." For other patients and families, or under other circumstances, it may be more appropriate to use the truth judiciously. The decision is not a simple one and, I submit, cannot be made according to a uniform rule or universal principle. The issue has been made much more difficult by the fact that less than full disclosure has been judged, at times, as malpractice.

The decisions of how much truth is called for or is appropriate, like the question of how much treatment is appropriate, should reflect the physician's fullest understanding of the patient's life rather than society's current attitudes about paternalism and truth telling.

Mr. N and his wife had shared a long life. They had faced suffering and danger, took risks, and had undoubtedly made many difficult choices. They shared a "microculture" that few outsiders could ever fully appreciate. It would have been presumptuous for me to believe that I could judge what might be best for my patient when the time arrived for telling Mr. N the "truth." At the time, however, I felt that it was a choice of whose wishes or needs—those of my patient or those of his wife—took precedence.

In fact, the very question "Whose needs?" reveals the central issue. As I see it now, the real dichotomy was between the needs of Mr. N *and* his wife, on the one hand, and my own need to adhere to a broad injunction that physicians have a responsibility to tell the truth to patients, on the other. This particular situation is not unique in medicine. Patients and physicians experience disease differently. Patients experience *illness* as a unique, personal, idiosyncratic event. Physicians understand *disease* in relation to a systematic body of information and a variable familiarity by experience.

This difference in perspective must always be bridged. Physicians who are viewed as "humanistic" or "holistic" recognize the epistemic chasm and, calling upon their empathic qualities, are able to bridge the gap to a greater or lesser degree. The patient and the patient's family must be considered in decision-making and in the truth telling that goes into making therapeutic and life-altering choices.

When one or several family members move beyond the usual role as interested, loving relatives to assume a role as "family caregiver," they have, in effect, a hybrid role. It is this role that poses unique challenges for both the physician and the patient. The physician is challenged to redefine who is being cared for. The aphorism that the physician cares for the "whole family" seems glib and oversimplified. The burden that family caregiving places on family members cannot escape the physician's attention. For the patient dependence on family members for care can bring to the surface painful issues reflecting family relationships that long antedate the family caregiving arrangement.

A Judicious Use of Paternalism

When I was a medical student and house officer and during the early years of my medical practice, the prevailing dictum (or so I believed) was that the truth should be used judiciously, as with any treatment administered by the physician. Patients rarely questioned the actions of their physicians. The word *cancer* was rarely spoken and patients usually were told that radiation treatments, hormones, or chemotherapeutic drugs were given to "prevent problems."

The prevailing notion today is very different. *Paternalism* has been rejected in favor of *patient autonomy* and the view that "full disclosure" is a requisite for good medical practice. Greatly increased patient awareness of sophisticated issues regarding diagnostic and treatment aspects of many illnesses is in part responsible for this dramatic change in the physician-patient relationship. In no small degree this shift can also be traced to the climate of fear of malpractice actions in medicine today.

Today most physicians would argue that patients should be "fully informed." Despite (or perhaps because of) its Latin root in the word *pater,* or *father,* paternalism has become an anathema. The potential risks or side effects of every treatment, no matter how unlikely, are described in considerable detail before obtaining the patient's consent. When such warnings are affixed to cigarette packs or bottles of alcohol, the intent is to discourage smoking by everyone and alcohol consumption by pregnant women. Yet, when the patient with intractable angina is advised that coronary angiography or angioplasty may lead to an arterial embolus, the loss of a limb, or emergency coronary bypass surgery, the intent is not to discourage the patient from undergoing the procedure. Nor can it can be honestly claimed that the recitation of this litany of possible disastrous complications is intended to give the patient the opportunity to make an "informed judgment."

Although this information is always presented in the guise of full disclosure and truth telling, the underlying motive has more to do with "documentation." Patients are generally not given the choice of whether they wish to hear all of the potential hazards of the procedure they are about to undergo! It has been suggested that this truth telling and informed consent be witnessed by a third party or even videotaped. The motive behind this routine practice is not simple, but truth telling and full disclosure are the norm in relations between patients and physicians today and in my view reflect a serious breakdown in this relationship.

I do not feel the same need to detail all the potential complications of a procedure or treatment that I have advised for my patient as do the consulting invasive cardiologist or the consulting oncologist to whom they have been referred. I can hear my reader murmuring, critically, "Paternalism, paternalism." Reflecting on my own life and medical encounters of members of my family, I am not sure that I am ready to reject a measure of paternalism. Our society cannot and should not return to the time, not very long ago, when patients were told very little and were expected to listen to the advice of a physician, "who knew best."

I do, however, think something important has been lost when a physician feels that every doubt and concern, however remote, unlikely, or frightening, must be shared with the patient. This form of presenting the "whole truth" to the patient bears a striking resemblance to the manner in which the *Physicians' Desk Reference* (*PDR*) lists all the potential side effects of every drug. While this comprehensive listing may be appropriate for the *PDR* (and I have some doubts about this), I surely do not feel that the physician should "reveal all" in the same way as a package insert. "Truth" and "facts" are not discrete, defined entities, like so many colored marbles, to be handed to the patient to accept or reject.

The case of Mr. and Mrs. N has led me to think through and alter to some degree my ideas about truth telling and the relationship of a physician to family caregivers. Physicians can learn from such challenges to accepted practices. Listening to patients and their family caregivers is a good place to start.

ACKNOWLEDGMENT

My earlier discussion of this case was published as "The Whole Truth...?" in Jerome Lowenstein, M.D., *The Midnight Meal and Other Essays about Doctors, Patients, and Medicine* (New Haven: Yale University Press, 1997), 76–80.

Part II / Home Care
Past and Present

CHAPTER FOUR

Family Caregiving in New England

Nineteenth-Century Community Care Gives Way to Twentieth-Century Institutions

Sheila M. Rothman

Caregiving takes place throughout the life cycle. Much of the care that is given as death nears reflects historical attitudes and practices. These practices reflect both family values and religious beliefs and, in ways that are less well known and understood, also reflect cultural assumptions about caregiving which have been established in social and health policies. These public pronouncements and practices have, in many instances, created remarkable and ongoing tensions between care privately given within the family and care publicly supported within an institution.

In the American context the general practice in social policy well into the nineteenth century was to rely in most, albeit not all, circumstances upon the family.* In case of illness it was the family's duty to nurse and nurture. Only

---

*There are very few studies that focus directly on the priority of family caregiving in the nineteenth century. See, for example, Abel 2001. On the obligations of family, see also Ruggles 1987. The first graduates of nursing schools generally cared for the sick and dying in their own homes. See S. Rothman 1978, 87-89. Histories of nursing also provide information on how the profession buttressed family caregiving (Reverby 1987). There are also numerous letters, diaries, and memoirs that document the reliance on family caregiving.

those who lacked a family—and in the nineteenth century *family* was defined in extended and communal terms—were to be cared for through public means, in a shack or jail if they were "furiously mad" or in an almshouse if they were strangers or very poor and debilitated by disease. Whether the institutions were funded through religious organizations or states and municipalities, they were intended to serve the "other," that is, outsiders to the society. For the insiders it was family, first, last, and always (D. Rothman 1971; Rosenberg 1987).

Caregiving Practices in Nineteenth-Century New England

As a result of these assumptions and practices, in the nineteenth century caregiving was an extraordinary burden, so all-consuming that it set the parameters of all women's lives, whether the women were married, single, or widowed (Ryan 1981; Cott 1977). For example, the obligation of Protestant women who lived in New England in the first half of the nineteenth century to care for their own children was so sacrosanct that, even when they themselves were sick and debilitated by disease, they were still expected to continue to oversee the physical and spiritual well-being of their children (S. Rothman 1994). Female kin were also obligated to care for sick family members.

This obligation took many different forms. Women, particularly single women, were expected to travel to the home of a sick relative to assist with caregiving (Chambers-Schiller 1984). These women often moved from home to home to provide assistance as it was needed. "My husband," one New England invalid woman explained to a friend in 1836, "has a maiden cousin about fifty years old, a Miss Stearns who is visiting me this term; she has no real home and stays around among friends and assists them." Single women made it possible for married women with a chronic illness to remain at home. "I think," the writer continued in a self-deprecating manner, "useful single women are the salt of the earth. What would become of us if everyone was married? I am sure all the invalid wives would soon be sold for rags" (qtd. in S. Rothman 1994, 97).

Caregiving was both a familial and communal effort in New England communities. Extended family members, including aunts, uncles, and cousins, were expected in times of crisis to provide care for sick and dying family members either in their own homes or in the homes of the sick for extended periods of time (Abel 1995). For women who did not have extended families or could not afford domestic help, communal organizations assumed responsibility. If the disease was chronic, the obligations persisted for years and even decades.

Take, for example, the case of consumption, as tuberculosis was called in this era before Robert Koch introduced the germ theory. The disease was understood to be hereditary and noncontagious. Unlike earlier epidemics that had ravaged Europe, consumption did not suddenly appear, devastate a population, and then abruptly recede (Park 1985). Its course was at once less precipitous and more tenacious, taking a grim toll year after year. Its sufferers did not succumb within a matter of days. Instead, acute attacks alternated with remissions. Since the process of wasting and dying could take a few years or span several decades, ministering to the sick and assisting them in fulfilling their domestic obligations often required the caregiving efforts of a network of kin (Sweester 1836).*

Men and women who contracted the disease remained at home and at times of crisis were cared for first and foremost by family and kin. To try to restore health, physicians frequently recommended that persons with consumption change climate and lifestyle. But, because the sick were expected to be cared for within the family, those with consumption followed this prescription by traveling to the homes of relatives in distant towns or rural areas and convalescing there for months. Kin were also expected to board the children of sick relatives. In the event the parents died, family members, including extended family members, assumed responsibility for the physical and spiritual care of the orphans (S. Rothman 1994, 1–24).

Since premature death from consumption was quite common, caring for the chronically ill and later for their orphan children affected the substance of women's lives (Leavitt 1986). Demographic data confirm this point.[†] The birth and death statistics of one town—Amherst, Massachusetts—for a single year, 1844, reveal the burden that caring for women who contracted consumption placed on all women. In 1844 Amherst had 2,550 residents, and in that year the town clerk recorded 61 births and 51 deaths. Of the 51 deaths

---

*There are many medical textbooks that describe the course of the disease and its chronicity. See, for example, Sweester 1836.

[†]Tuberculosis was the leading cause of death in the United States during the first half of the nineteenth century, responsible for almost 25 percent of all deaths. See Shattuck 1948, 94.

14, or more than 1 out of 4, were from consumption. Although the ages of those who died from the disease ranged from nine to eighty-four, half of all the women who died were married women between the ages of twenty-seven and fifty (S. Rothman 1994, 95).

By linking this demographic data to the obligations that consumption conferred on family and community, the extent of caregiving obligations is apparent. Given the course of the disease and the way it wasted the bodies of those who contracted it, many of the women who died in 1844 would not have been physically able to manage their domestic and child-rearing responsibilities for several years before their deaths. Each would have required, and received, the sustained assistance of family and friends. If the invalid women could not afford domestic help, the sewing circle would repair their clothing, and friends and neighbors would supply meals and provide nursing. When the invalids became incapacitated, an unmarried sister or cousin or perhaps a widowed mother or aunt would move into the household. As death neared and the invalid became still further debilitated, the obligations of family and community to provide care for the sick and those they cared for would have become still greater. Indeed, the "intensive care" given in a New England family was not provided by a machine monitored by strangers but, rather, was bestowed in the home of the chronically ill by a network of female family members, friends, and neighbors. The level of care intensified as the illness progressed, often reaching a crescendo as death neared (S. Rothman 1994, 116–27).

In New England all caregiving responsibilities were reciprocal, buttressed and defended by social expectations and religious precepts. New England families shared an Evangelical Christian faith with a series of religious precepts that clearly set out the obligations of the sick to the healthy and the healthy to the sick. These families lived in close-knit and highly interdependent communities in which numerous church-based mutual assistance organizations provided material assistance, nursing care, and spiritual support to the chronically ill (Rosenberg 1985; Brown 1987).

The social implications of the New England caregiving ethos and practices became apparent when a mother with consumption set out rules of proper comportment for her children. These rules were laid down with the knowledge that her children would soon become orphans. Deborah Fiske, whose mother had died from consumption when she was two years old and had been raised in the homes of family members, warned her five-year-old daughter, Helen, of the necessity of obedience. When Deborah had an acute attack and was not able to care for her daughter, Helen was sent for an extended visit to the home of an aunt who was likely to become her guardian. In her daily letters to Helen, Deborah, in a very pedagogic manner, stressed the need for cheerful submission. "I hope you will be very happy ... and try every day to make them as little trouble as possible. Remember that it is a great deal for them to put you to bed every night and help dress you every morning and prepare your food and answer your questions." Deborah told Helen that there were many things she could do to repay her aunt's kindness: "You can dust chairs, and take the lamps down from the chambers, and carry away dishes." Knowing that this was a trial visit, Deborah continued: "There are some things you must be careful to avoid doing, and I shall print them on separate lines that you may notice every one. Never talk when others present are speaking[.] Never occupy the rocking chair or the easiest chair in a room when any older person is present... Never speak of hating things or people[.] Never say you do not love what is placed before you."

Thus, rules of behavior which mothers often repeated casually to their children became imperatives that a mother living in the shadow of death warned her children not to violate. Instructing a five-year-old that she should "never leave chairs out of place or push them up against the paper...when you set them away" was not testimony to a fetish about good manners but reflected the power, even the tyranny, which reciprocal obligations held over both the sick and the healthy. In this case disobedience, willfulness, or carelessness might sever the ties that Deborah had so carefully constructed to protect Helen's moral and spiritual well-being (S. Rothman 1994, 95).

The importance of reciprocal obligations became even more apparent as death neared. The dying person became the focus of familial attention. She summoned those to whom she wished to say a last good-bye. No one refused, even if it meant taking a several-day-long stagecoach ride in the middle of a New England winter. The dying person also chose those she wanted to watch over her and to pray and sing with her as she waited for her final call. In return she gave the watchers' gifts, tokens of affection, which symbolized the continuity between the living and the dead.

The same dynamic is also evident in the experiences of New England men who had consumption. Far more often than women, men tried to fulfill the optimal medical prescription by traveling to a mild climate to restore health. This frequently meant booking a passage on a packet ship going south in the fall and returning home in late May. Away from their families and the New England institutions that bounded their lives, the men clustered together and made surrogate families out of casual acquaintances, so as to carry out their social and religious obligations.

On the Caribbean island of St. Croix, New England men boarded in the few houses near the harbor. They visited one another, nursed one another, watched over and prayed for one another, and, as a last duty, wrote to the family of the courage and serenity with which husband or son had faced his final trial. "Before this trembles in your hand," Samuel Weston informed the wife of one consumptive in 1819, "every symptom warrants that probability that the man you have held so dear will be with us no more." He went on to assure her: "Death with him had no terrors for he firmly believed he would be admitted to the mansions of the blessed" (qtd. in S. Rothman 1994, 62).

The very intensity of these obligations also explains attitudes toward caretaking institutions and toward those who became the objects of care within them. Institutions for persons labeled deviant and dependent were viewed by Protestant New England families as a last resort. Even as nineteenth-century asylum superintendents urged families to put their members under their care as early in the disease as possible, the families did not comply. They would only institutionalize those who became disturbed beyond control. Only very manic persons, those with extensive delusions or melancholia, entered the asylum. It took an extreme manifestation of disease to justify having strangers—that is, those who were not family or friends—provide caregiving for chronically ill kin (Tomes 1994).

The Dominance of Public Caregiving in the Twentieth Century

The paradigm of care which held in the early nineteenth century underwent a fundamental change at the beginning of the twentieth century. This change persisted, without any significant challenges, into the 1960s. At this time institutional care took on an unprecedented significance and legitimacy. The stigma of institutionalized care for the chronically ill and dying declined markedly, and family obligations were redefined in ways that justified using the resources of caretaking institutions. A list of these institutions by type confirms the point. They included hospitals for persons with mental illness, state schools for retarded children, sanatoriums for persons with tuberculosis, and nursing homes for frail and elderly persons (D. Rothman 1980).

Why did this shift in attitudes toward institutional care occur? To some degree innovations in medical technology initiated and then further encouraged the shift. The experiences of persons with tuberculosis who became patients in sanatoriums in the first decades of the twentieth century exemplify the dynamics of the change and its impact on the sick and their caregivers. Their experiences are particularly revealing because the structure of the facility, its regimen, and patient-caretaker relationships were in every way antithetical to the ideals of caregiving which marked the life cycle of New England families.

A new medical understanding of the etiology and course of tuberculosis was partly responsible for this dramatic reordering of caregiving responsibilities. Departments of Health, aware of the contagious nature of the disease and the threat it posed to the healthy, promulgated regulations to confine those with the disease, even against their will. The fear of contagion became all the more widespread because tuberculosis was no longer a disease of all (as it had been in the nineteenth century) but a disease of some—mainly the poor and immigrants. Thus, principles of bacteriology more generally and the epidemiology of tuberculosis more specifically led directly to the construction of a network of sanatoria. These new facilities were designed to promote societal well-being by isolating the sick and to encourage individual well-being by ostensibly implementing a therapeutic regimen (Caldwell 1988).

Given this framework, sanatoria were often constructed in isolated rural settings. Their location, generally distant from the city and even railroad depots, and their mission, to protect and cure, made them inaccessible to friends and family. Visiting hours were carefully controlled and extremely limited. The shared values, strong religious faith, integration of the sick into the community, and interlocking obligations between the sick and the healthy which characterized caregiving relationships in New England disappeared inside the sanatorium (Bates 1992).

In the sanatorium strangers—that is, doctors and nurses—replaced family and friends as caregivers. The medical mission that linked confinement to cure buttressed the authority of the staff as it diminished the importance of intimacy with family and friends. It also legitimized institutional care and encouraged families to send those with the symptoms of the disease to the sanatorium.

Yet what society defined as a public health crusade, the sick experienced as confinement and stigmatization. As one patient put it: "If a criminal thinks he is the only social outcast, let him take heart. There are some of us without blemish or without breaking a law of society that are still as much of an outcast as he who robbed or murdered. One enters a jail; the other enters a sanatorium. Each comes out 'branded for life'" (S. Rothman 1994, 229). From the patients' perspective entering the sanatorium was like making a pact with the devil, sacrificing dignity in return for the promise of prolonged life and perhaps restored health.

In the sanatorium numerous rules and regulations enhanced medical authority and distanced patients from caregivers. The values inherent in family caregiving were deprecated in the sanatorium. Knowledge replaced familiarity; authority replaced compassion. As persons with tuberculosis confronted one of the most challenging periods of their lives, they were forced to do so without the comfort of family and friends. As ties with families weakened, patients often became bitter and bereft. "During my first few months," one of them recalled, "I tried as far as possible to hold myself aloof from my surroundings ... It was impossible, however, to maintain this detached attitude for the ties binding me to the life I had left were gradually loosened. At first I had many letters from my friends...[but] their forgetfulness...forced me to thrust reluctant roots into this alien soil." Or, as another put it after a few months, stories about family from home seemed "like talk about people long dead. The only real things were connected to the sanatorium. The only real people, the other patients, the doctors, the nurses" (qtd. in S. Rothman 1994, 234–35).

Death was a taboo topic in the sanitorium. The staff was so convinced of the curative potential of the sanatorium regimen that they were unwilling to acknowledge the fact that deaths occurred or even to admit that patients died. Instead, they contended that, if patients cheerfully complied with a regimen of diet and rest, they would be cured. This conviction permeated the rule books that patients received when they were admitted to the sanatorium and the therapeutic regimen. "Getting well depends on the patient," one rule book declared. "Rest, fresh air, good food...all help. But if the patient does not have the will power, the honesty, the character, to obey the rules nothing will save him. Getting well depends on you" (MacDonald 1948, 72–73).

The rhetoric of willpower served many purposes. Patient compliance simplified the job of the staff. The rhetoric also shifted the responsibility for failing to achieve a cure from the staff to the patients. It was the patients' lack of discipline, not the inadequacy of the regimen, which was to blame. In this spirit the staff maintained that, when untoward events occurred, the rules alone would be adequate to keep up the patients' morale, even when—and the rest of the sentence was left unsaid—they witnessed the deaths of other patients (S. Rothman 1994, 233).

Yet death did occur in the sanatorium. The fact that it occurred and was not discussed frustrated the patients. Thus, when a group of patients learned that a young man who had scrupulously followed the rules "threw a hemorrhage" and died, one patient noted that "he cured better than anyone in the whole place." "I know it," another patient agreed. "And some of these guys that chase around and get drunk, play the women, sneak out late at night—they get along all right. It makes you wonder" (McClintock 1931, 214).

Thus, every time a patient died, the tension between the staff and patients mounted. Some patients would leave the facility against medical advice. Others would decide that there was no point in following the rules. Living on the edge, they might just as well do what they pleased. Why die without ever having lived? So, whether they remained or left, in one way or another, the unwillingness of the staff to acknowledge or discuss death led patients to subvert medical authority (S. Rothman 1994, 241).

Whatever frustrations patients experienced in caregiving institutions and whatever remorse families expressed, institutional confinement became integral to health policy in the first half of the twentieth century. Sociologists list numerous reasons for the widespread acceptance of institutional care. They include smaller families that did not have the resources to provide family caregiving as well as the general secularization of the society. What is often neglected in these analyses is medical legitimation. The authority of physicians and medicine was so elevated that the prospect of cure, even for those for whom a cure seemed most remote, became an acceptable reason for indefinite confinement in a caregiving institution. Examples abound. In the 1950s physicians urged parents with retarded children to send these children to an institution. Whatever the deficits in nursing or education, medical supervision and medical authority justified their isolation (Rothman and Rothman 1984). Some observers noted the psychological cost to both patients and families. In 1897 the renowned physician William Osler called attention to the

indifference, even disdain, for family caregiving which health care professionals displayed.

> The tender mother, the loving wife, the devoted sister, the faithful friend, and the
> old servant who ministered to his wants and carried out the doctor's instructions
> so far as they were consistent with the sick man's wishes—all, all are gone; these
> old familiar faces; and now you reign supreme, and have added to every illness a
> domestic complication of which our fathers knew nothing. You have upturned
> an inalienable right in displacing those whom I have just mentioned. You are in-
> truders, innovators, and usurpers, dislocating as you do, from their tenderest and
> most loving duties these mothers, wives and sisters. (Hinohara 1993, 639)

But, although Osler's pronouncements on clinical medicine were never vio-
lated, his admonitions on the problems that emerged as hospital personnel
usurped the responsibilities of families to care for persons near the end of life
were ignored.

As the medical staff assumed the obligations of family to care for those near
the end of life, they also banished family members from the bedside. David
Sudnow, a sociologist who observed caretaking practices on the wards of general hospitals during the 1960s, noted the strategies the staff used to maintain
a distance between dying persons and their families. When patients were in
critical condition, Sudnow noted, they "theoretically have the right to round-
the-clock visitors." But in the institutions he studied the "nurses strive to separate relatives from patients about to die...They urge family members to go
home and await further news there, or insist that they wait outside in the cor-
ridors and not in the patient's room." Why? If relative were present, then "a
more constant vigilance over the patient's condition must be maintained, requiring in effect the removal of a nurse from other activities to spend exclusive time at the bedside." This was considered both inefficient and futile.
Physicians shared these attitudes. They too preferred "that relatives be kept
away from the bedside of the dying patient, so that he [the doctor] is freer to
leave the bedside himself and attend to other matters" (Sudnow 1967, 80–81).

Nothing could be farther from the values of caregiving in New England
families than Sudnow's observations of a nurse who spent several minutes trying to close the eyelids of a dying patient. "This involved," he noted, "slowly
but somewhat forcefully pushing the two lids together to get them to adhere
in a closed position." When Sudnow questioned her, the nurse explained, "A

patient's eyelids are always closed after death, so that the body will resemble a sleeping person." After death, she reported, "it was more difficult to accomplish a complete lid closure, especially after the body muscles have begun to tighten and the eyelids become less pliable, more resistant, and have a tendency to move apart...She always tried, she reported, to close them before death while the eyes were still elastic and more easily manipulated. This allowed ward personnel to more quickly wrap the body upon death...and was considerate, she pointed out, of those who preferred to handle dead bodies as little as possible" (Sudnow 1967, 66). And what was common in the general hospital in the 1960s became amplified in the intensive care unit in the 1970s and 1980s. It was no longer the nurse but the machine that monitored the dying process (Zussman 1992).

Even as Sudnow was writing, caretaker institutions had began to lose some of their standing. Their authority challenged by class action lawsuits, new pharmaceuticals (such as psychotropic drugs and antibacterials), and the anti-institutional ethos of the era (Rothman and Rothman 1984, 106–24). Nevertheless, policies have not been put in place which buttress family values and promote family caregiving. Although I cannot fully trace these changes, let me give a few examples. State schools for developmentally disabled persons and state institutions for mentally ill persons have been closed, but the resources that would enable families to care for their relatives at home are minimal. Nursing homes are institutions of last resort, but funds for home health care are not widely available. And, as more aging women remain at home alone, they become more physically and mentally frail. A new and terrifying diagnosis—"found at home"—in which a woman is found either unable to call for help or dead—points to the inadequacies of our health care priorities (Gurley et al. 1996).

Hospice, and the spirit of hospice, has offered one important alternative. It provides a way for families to be at the bedside without the extraordinary burdens that were assumed by New England women. Nevertheless, more attention and funding need to be devoted to devising models of care throughout the life cycle—models that appreciate the strengths and limitations of caretaking institutions and the needs of families. Until this is achieved, many Americans will be forced to rely on caretaking institutions that have lost their legitimacy and which deliver less than optimal care. Put most succinctly, we have to do better.

REFERENCES

Abel, Emily K. (2001). *Hearts of Wisdom: American Women Caring for Kin: 1850–1940*. Cambridge: Harvard University Press.

———. (1995). "'Man, Woman and Chore Boy': Transformations in the Antagonistic Demands of Work and Care on Women in the Nineteenth and Twentieth Centuries." *Milbank Quarterly* 73:187–211.

Bates, Barbara. (1992). *Bargaining for Life: A Social History of Tuberculosis, 1876–1939*. Philadelphia: University of Pennsylvania Press.

Brown, Irene Quenzler. (1987). "Death, Friendship, and Female Identity during New England's Second Great Awakening." *Journal of Family History* (12):367–87.

Caldwell, Mark. (1988). *The Last Crusade: The War on Consumption, 1862–1954*. New York: Atheneum.

Chambers-Schiller, Lee Virginia. (1984). *Liberty, a Better Husband: Single Women in America: The Generations of 1780–1840*. New Haven: Yale University Press.

Cott, Nancy. (1977). *The Bonds of Womanhood: "Woman's Sphere" in New England, 1780–1835*. New Haven: Yale University Press.

Gurley R. J., et al. (1996). "Persons Found in Their Homes Helpless or Dead." *New England Journal of Medicine* 334:1710–16.

Hinohara, Shigeaki. (1993). "Sir William Osler's Philosophy on Death." *Annals of Internal Medicine* 118:638–42.

Leavitt, Judith Walzer. (1986). *Brought to Bed: Child-Bearing in America, 1750–1950*. New York: Oxford University Press.

MacDonald, Betty. (1948). *The Plague and I*. Philadelphia: J. B. Lippincott.

McClintock, Marshall. (1931). *We Take to Bed*. New York: Jonathan Cape and Harrison Smith.

Park, Katharine. (1985). *Doctors and Medicine in Early Renaissance Florence*. (Princeton, N.J.: Princeton University Press.

Reverby, Susan M. (1987). *Ordered to Care: The Dilemma of American Nursing, 1850–1945*. New York: Cambridge University Press.

Rosenberg, Carroll-Smith. (1985). "The Female World of Love and Ritual: Relations between Women in Nineteenth-Century America." In *Disorderly Conduct: Visions of Gender in Victorian America*, ed. Carroll-Smith Rosenberg. New York: Alfred A. Knopf.

Rosenberg, Charles E. (1987). *The Care of Strangers: The Rise of America's Hospital System*. New York: Basic Books.

Rothman, David J. (1971). *The Discovery of the Asylum: Order and Disorder in the New Republic*. Boston: Little, Brown.

———. (1980). *Conscience and Convenience: The Asylum and Its Alternatives in Progressive America*. Boston: Little, Brown.

Rothman, David J., and Sheila M. Rothman. (1984). *The Willowbrook Wars: A Decade of Struggle for Social Justice*. New York: Harper and Row.

Rothman, Sheila M. (1978). *Woman's Proper Place: A History of Changing Ideals and Practices, 1870 to the Present*. New York: Basic Books.

———. (1994). *Living in the Shadow of Death: Tuberculosis and the Social Experience of Illness in American History*. New York: Basic Books.

Ruggles, Steven. (1987). *Prolonged Connections: The Rise of the Extended Family in Nineteenth Century England and America*. Madison: University of Wisconsin Press.

Ryan, Mary P. (1981). *Cradle of the Middle Class: The Family in Oneida County, New York, 1790–1865*. Cambridge: Cambridge University Press.

Shattuck, Lemuel. (1948). *Report of the Sanitary Commission of Massachusetts*. Cambridge Mass.: Harvard University Press.

Sudnow, David. (1967). *Passing On*. Englewood Cliffs, N.J.: Prentice-Hall.

Sweester, William. (1836). *Treatise on Consumption*. Boston: T. H. Carter.

Tomes, Nancy. (1984). *Generous Confidence: Thomas Story Kirkbride and the Art of Asylum Keeping, 1840–1883*. New York: Cambridge University Press.

Zussman, Robert. (1992). *Intensive Care: Medical Ethics and the Medical Profession*. Chicago: University of Chicago Press.

CHAPTER FIVE

Nurses and Their Changing Relationship to Family Caregivers

Mathy Mezey

While most people expect to care for an ill spouse, parent, or child at some point in their lives, typically they envision that caregiving will be short-lived—during recovery from an acute illness, following surgery, or at the end of life. Frequently, however, family members find themselves providing care over years or decades. Whatever the specific circumstances, most family caregivers do not expect to provide care alone. They anticipate practical and emotional help from kinfolk and friends. In cases of serious illness they look for the active involvement of health care professionals, and the person they often think will be most responsive to their needs is a nurse.

Family caregivers and nurses are, at least in theory, natural allies. Family caregivers need the services that nurses are trained to provide. Nurses are taught that their mission is to help patients recover from an illness and, if possible, regain functional independence. Family members are an essential part of that care. Anecdotal impressions and surveys, such as satisfaction data from patients and families, indicate that family caregivers in general are highly satisfied with the help they get from nurses.

Nevertheless, there is substantial evidence that all is not well in this relationship. Family caregivers report inadequate care or negative experiences with nurses: incompetent care, impersonal care, too little care, or no care. Similarly, nurses are quick to cite family members as impeding their ability to provide care to patients. In one hospital, when surveyed, nurses named "difficult" family members as their biggest "problem." To some degree this may be seen as a manifestation of the different cultures of nursing and family.

The purpose of this chapter is to explore this relationship, focusing primarily on nurses and family caregivers for elderly people and adults with chronic illness. Nursing refers to professional registered nurses (RNs) and master's degree–prepared advanced practice nurses (APNs). This chapter begins with a historical perspective, then looks at the current status of nursing practice related to family caregiving, and closes with an analysis of what we may expect in the future. The analysis demonstrates that the natural alliance between nursing and family caregivers has been weakened by nursing's dependency on the predominant cultures of medicine and, more recently, regulation and economics. Yet the basic reasons for the alliance still exist and can be nurtured.

The Professionalization of Nursing and the Dominance of Hospital Care

Given today's emphasis on home care agencies, it is important to keep in mind that throughout the nineteenth century families provided virtually all the care to infirm relatives in their own or the relative's home. Family members may have engaged a neighbor or servant to assist in the caregiving chores. Apart from tuberculosis, as described by Sheila Rothman in Chapter 4, most illnesses were short-lived and acute. Patients suffered from primary infections, such as diphtheria or pneumonia, or infections arising from trauma or tissue injury.

In the late 1800s well-to-do families began to hire "trained nurses" to assist a family member in providing care. These nurses were hired by and reported directly to the family. Physicians often recommended their preferred nurses, who moved from case to case. In the home nurses assisted rather than replaced family caregivers, often taking night shifts. Because most jobs were obtained through word of mouth, nurses' initial and subsequent employment was very dependent on the good relationships they developed with families.

Poor families caring for a sick relative at home in the late 1800s were aided by the development of visiting nurses deployed by public agencies and private groups into homes. These nurses realized that, because they visited only episodically, the family had to maintain primary responsibility for delivering care. Thus, visiting and home care nurses saw one of their primarily responsibilities as teaching family members to manage their sick relative's health problems.

Only with the growth of hospitals and the move of trained nurses into hospitals in the early twentieth century did families trust professional nurses to substitute for the caregiving function of the family (Lynaugh 1996, 73). Admonished by professionals that patients recovered best in hospitals that were clean, calm and orderly, families ceded their caregiving responsibilities to the nursing staff. Families were relegated to "visitor" status and allowed access to patients at designated and limited hours. Families reclaimed the patient when he or she died, which was frequently the case, or when the patient was discharged home after a long stay. Thus, as hospitals became accepted as institutions for the sick and the dying, the need for the family to provide care was substantially altered and diminished.

With hospital ascendancy in management of the sick and with the shift in the location of care of the sick, the home health care delivery system became somewhat marginalized (Rinke and Holt 2000). Nurses delivered home health care only under a physician's order and only after the physician had seen the patient, typically in his office or the hospital.

Despite the migration of large number of nurses away from home care into hospitals, public health nursing continued to attract the "best and the brightest" in nursing. Public health, including home care, epitomized modern nursing: management of complex health needs, independent assessment and decision making, and the opportunity to teach and work with the patient and family over an extended period of time. A nurse was required to have one year of hospital experience in order to work in public health or home care. The autonomy and authority that characterized home care nursing is evident in programs such as the New York City Department of Health's protocol for premature babies. These infants could not be released from the hospital until a visiting nurse reported that the family was prepared and that the home was safe.

Several factors occurred in the mid- to late 1960s which made hospitals the preferred work environment for nurses. Of great importance was the introduction of technology such as respirators and intravenous (IV) pumps and the creation of intensive care units (ICUs). Because the treatment of ICU patients was complex, ICUs required nurses with advanced skills. Nursing education began to prepare these nurses. New graduates saw the ICU as the site where they could fully use their scientific preparation: understanding the physiological consequences of the patient's condition, mastering complex technology, and identifying impending complications or downturns in the patient's condition. Because they were the health professionals on site twenty-four hours a day, ICU nurses had both independence and authority.

The advent of ICUs further separated family members from the care of the sick. In the name of science and the "miracles" achievable in ICUs, the perception by health care professionals that families were a problem was accentuated. While families might want to visit more frequently, professionals saw them as interfering with complex and technological medical care. By the 1970s and 1980s the women's movement and enlightened childcare practices had liberalized family visiting hours in maternity and pediatric units. But ICUs retained the view of families as bothersome "interlopers." Even today ICU visits are limited to five to fifteen minutes every hour or two hours.

In addition to ICUs, the development of new technologies and the ability to offer active and often complex treatment to patients stimulated further nursing specialization in hospitals. Management of extremely sick cardiac and cancer patients required nurses with exquisite clinical skills who could practice comfortably alongside physicians. Thus, in hospitals the focus of a nurse's practice shifted from a primary relationship with the patient and family to that of a primary relationship with the physician. As nurses sought to master technology and treatment regimens, family needs moved ever further from the center of nursing interest and responsibility. Nursing culture became more like physician culture, valuing scientific skill and technological know-how rather than communication and comfort.

As acute care became high-tech, the landscape of home care for nurses paled in contrast to the challenge of working in hospitals. Increasingly, patients admitted for acute care recuperated in the hospital or in "step-down" facilities. Acute care patients were almost fully recovered when they came home, with little need for dressings or technology. Thus, nurses felt that their newly acquired knowledge and technical skills were wasted in caring for patients at home. Home care increasingly became the practice of caring for elderly patients or for adult patients with chronic illness, clearly not the preferred work environment for a highly educated young nurse.

One conclusion that can be drawn from this brief review is that a professionalized, scientific, and institutionally based culture of nursing served to "crowd out" nursing's traditional attention to family. This, however, is only partially true. Individual nurses continued to feel strongly allied with families. They continued to define nurse caregiving interventions as focused on both the patient and the family. Yet, in an effort to be taken seriously as health care professionals and to define their practice as "evidence based," the nursing profession tended to overemphasize nursing actions and outcomes that were more easily quantified and measured and to underemphasize nursing actions for which outcomes were hard to measure. Until recently, outcomes related to family have tended to fall in the latter category. Some new areas of nursing investigation, described in the following pages, are beginning to reexamine nurses' involvement with families.

Current Status: Family Caregiving, Nursing, and Home Care

The enactment of federally funded Medicare and Medicaid in 1965 introduced the current era of home care nursing. Chapter 6 by Rick Surpin and Eileen Hanley and Chapter 7 by Judith Feder and Carol Levine, in this volume, provide more detail about Medicare. Although Medicare regulations apply only to its providers and beneficiaries—people over sixty-five, those with end-stage renal disease, and some people with disabilities—its policies have become benchmarks for most other kinds of insurance. For this chapter's focus on nursing it is important to recognize that Medicare totally realigned the incentives for a nurse's role in home care and, by so doing, changed the culture of nursing. Instead of focusing on the whole patient and family, nurses are paid to attend to a particular body part or disease entity. Many nurses had welcomed the prospect of strengthening home care in order to help patients and families cope with the residual of illnesses that up until that time had been addressed by longer recuperative periods in the hospital. But it has not worked out that way.

As B. Vladeck describes the advent of Medicare, "Home health care for the elderly was a relatively limited and novel idea in 1965, but the case was made, as it has been ever since, that organized home care services could reduce the length of inpatient hospital stays—the primary service for which the original

Medicare program was designed to pay" (2000, 232). Several changes occurred in the early 1980s. Medicare instituted a Prospective Payment System for hospitals that reimbursed hospitals by diagnosis-related groups (DRGs) rather than actual length of stay, giving hospitals a financial incentive to discharge patients sooner. Moreover, Congress opened the ranks of home care agencies to for-profit groups and eliminated a requirement for a prior hospitalization in order to receive home care benefits. In 1988 a federal judge ruled, in the case of *Duggan v. Bowen,* that the Health Care Financing Administration (HCFA, now called the Center for Medicare and Medicaid Services, or CMS) had failed to consider the intent of Congress—to expand home care services— in its administrative rules for home care. As a result, many HCFA regulations were dropped, for-profit home care agencies proliferated, especially in the South and West, and costs increased rapidly.

This uncontrolled expansion led to the Balanced Budget Act of 1997, which sharply reduced payments to home care agencies and tightened regulatory control. The rise of managed care and the advent of the Medicare Interim Payment system in the 1990s made it more difficult for home care agencies to receive authorization for home care services and severely limited their scope and duration (Stone 2001).

In home care, as a result of these regulatory and reimbursement changes, nurses have moved from their original role as helpers to and teachers of family caregivers to that of "pieceworkers" who focus on short-term, acute-care patient goals. Medicare-funded home care pays for post-acute, short-term services: short-term rehabilitation, management of conditions that have not resolved in the hospital, and teaching that quickly prepares patients and family caregivers to render care independently.

Family caregivers were seen as a revenue-neutral response to the forces causing health costs to soar: extended hospital stays, higher than anticipated use of home care, and the exorbitant overall costs of long-term care. More and more patients with complex health care needs were returned home early in their stage of recuperation or remained at home rather than being admitted to the hospital at all (Arras and Dubler 1996). At the same time, the patients' rights movement advocated policies that maximized patient "autonomy" and the patient's right to decide their plan of care, a perspective that was reinforced by the demands of young men with AIDS who insisted that their preferred site of care was the home.

Unfortunately, the imperative to return the responsibility of providing home care to families failed to take into account the substantial changes that patients and families had undergone since the early decades of the twentieth century, when families last were called on to serve as primary caregivers. Patients were now much older than in the first half of the 1900s, and their illnesses were chronic, multidimensional, and complex. Caregiving situations were highly diverse: cancer, AIDS, cardiovascular disease, diabetes, and dementia. The regimens that constituted the patient's plan of care required complex medication schedules and treatments and often the use of complex technology. Families were thus being asked to provide care unassisted in situations requiring substantial clinical skills that lay people, especially those new to the caregiving role, do not have (Arras and Dubler 1996; Levine 2000; Schumacher, Stewart, and Archbold 2000).

Societal demands that families assume responsibility for caregiving were also at odds with the marked changes in families over the last fifty years. Although family members do provide the bulk of home care, the number of women in the workforce, delayed childbearing, divorce and remarriage, and the tendency of family members to live in different parts of the country placed severe restrictions on the ability of family members to meet caregiving responsibilities. Family caregivers often faced simultaneous competing demands of work, childcare, and the welfare of several aged relatives, each of which required substantial assistance with care.

Similar to families, the nursing profession has also undergone substantial changes. Most nurses working today have never actually provided care in a patient's home, either as a student or as a graduate nurse. The overwhelming majority of nurses (80 percent) work in hospitals. With patients now staying an average of only six days in hospitals, nurses in hospitals have few opportunities to teach and prepare families for care at home (Health Forum 2000). Of the nation's 2.2 million professional nurses (RNs) only 17 percent (408,000 nurses) work in community and public health centers. In a time of a nursing shortage, as is the current situation, nurses prefer to work in hospitals as compared to home care or long-term care settings.

Moreover, a review of textbooks and syllabi suggests that academic nursing programs teach very little content about family caregiving needs. In reviewing nursing textbooks for end-of-life care issues, Ferrell (2001) found, for example, that family was not mentioned in 71 percent of textbooks reviewed. Although professional nursing educational programs profess to focus their instruction on patients and families, there is very little information about how these programs prepare nurses to work at home or with family caregivers. Content on family caregiving is hard to track because it is not taught in a separate course but is, instead, integrated into many courses.

In addition to professional nurses prepared with a baccalaureate or associate degree, there are currently over 400,000 specialty nurses, those certified by the American Nurses Credentialing Center (ANCC) and other professional certifying organizations. Over 80 academic masters programs prepare advanced practice nurses (APN) for specialization in areas such as family, adult, pediatric, and geriatric nursing. Between 1991 and 1999, 24,400 advanced practice specialty nurses were prepared for family practice with patients across the life span. Programs that prepare family nurse practitioners (FNPs) are the only advanced practice nursing specialty that has required content on family caregiving. In addition to FNPs, an additional 70,000 nurses are certified by the ANCC as nurse practitioners and clinical nurse specialists in adult women's health and geriatrics. While almost all these nurse specialists care for older patients and their family members, the amount of content these practitioners receive in family caregiving is unknown. Community health advanced practice nursing programs rank fourth in enrollment behind pediatrics, adult medicine, and family medicine. Only about 400 nurses are ANCC certified as community health nurses. Six programs nationally prepare advanced practice nurses for practice in home care, and only 46 nurses are ANCC certified as advanced practice home health nurses (ANCC 1999).

Today over 7,500 Medicare- and Medicaid-certified Home Care Agencies (CHAs) serve 7.2 million people annually (NAHC 2000). In 1999 there were 252 million Medicare-certified home health visits, averaging 70 visits per patient use (each patient contact with a nurse, therapist, or other health care professional counts as a separate visit). Medicare and Medicaid home health expenditures now total $14.1 billion annually (HCFA 2000). Reimbursement by Medicare and other private insurance continues to focus the work of nurses in the home on short-term outcomes, with Medicare reimbursement tied to whether the patient needs "hands-on" care and services requiring "skilled nursing judgments." Thus, there is almost no incentive to assess the caregiving needs of family members or to teach family members how to provide care.

For an older person or for someone with a chronic illness, recuperation from an acute illness is often delayed or derailed by the patient's age and multiple chronic conditions, which are unrecognized under Medicare home care reimbursement. By forcing agencies to focus on short-term recuperative goals, Medicare reimbursement for home care has been a "trap" that has made it impossible to structure and focus nursing care adequately on patient, let alone family, caregiving needs. The lasting effect of Medicare funding on nursing culture is evident when you hear a home care nurse describe her role in terms of "units of work" and "reimbursable services" rather than patient and family caregiver needs.

Despite the programmatic and reimbursement obstacles that impede nurses' ability to work with family caregivers, there are some model programs that provide comprehensive care. While family caregivers are important adjuncts, these programs are based on the elder person as beneficiary; family caregivers are not their primary focus. The best known is the Program for All-Inclusive Care to the Elderly (PACE) for frail elders, which replicates the original On Lok program in San Francisco for dually eligible Medicare and Medicaid elders. Some other examples are the National Institutes of Health (NIH)–funded Transitional Care program and the Visiting Nurse Association of Philadelphia's Housecalls program.

Financing for most of these programs is either through full or partial Medicare and/or Medicaid capitation. Thus, these models benefit from financing that rewards working with patients and family caregivers in order to keep patients at home and avoid unnecessary hospitalization and nursing home placement. The model programs use advanced practice nurses, usually working in collaboration with physicians or with a team of health care providers. These models capitalize on the skills and inclinations of APNs to support family members in their role as caregivers. Since 1999 APNs are fully reimbursed under most health plans, including Medicare, to provide care to patients and family members. Unfortunately, they are also subject to the same financial constraints that impede physicians' ability to focus on family needs, including the constraints in home care.

Moving Forward: Family Caregiving, Nursing, and Home Care

Clearly, the current climate of health care provides reasons to be cautious in forecasting improvements in relationships between family caregivers and nurses. Nevertheless, there are some changes in nursing education and practice and in financing for home care which offer opportunities to strengthen relationships between family caregivers and professional nurses.

Strengthening family caregiver skills

There is a growing interest within nursing in helping to identify and strengthen family caregiving skills (Stewart et al. 2001; Schumacher et al. 1999). The concept of caregiving skills acknowledges that families are being called on to provide ever more complex care to ill relatives. Family caregivers provide care unassisted in situations requiring more clinical skill than should be expected of lay people, especially those new to the caregiving role. Family caregiving skills have been defined as the ability to engage effectively and smoothly in nine core caregiving processes (Schumacher et al. 1999):

1. Monitoring: keeping an eye on things
2. Interpreting: making sense of what is observed
3. Making decisions: choosing a course of action
4. Taking action: carrying out caregiving instructions
5. Providing hands-on care: carrying out medical and nursing procedures attending to both safety and comfort
6. Making adjustments: finding the "right" strategy
7. Accessing resources
8. Working together with the ill person: sensitivity to the personhood of the care receiver and caregiver
9. Negotiating the health system.

There is also a recognition that we know all too little about family caregivers' needs for help. In following older patients during a hospital stay and at home following their hospitalization, Naylor (1999) found that one in five family caregivers reported their own health as fair or poor. Very few of these caregivers had helped lift a sick relative, gotten them out of bed, or helped a sick person to walk or to use the telephone before the patient's current hospital stay. Half of the caregivers had provided no help to the relative at all prior to hospitalization.

Nursing education is moving to help family caregivers master day-to-day caregiving practices rather than only providing information.

Improving the health promotion activities of family caregivers

Nurses have also recently demonstrated an interest in helping family care-givers strengthen their own resources as a way to protect them from the stress of caregiving (Given and Given 1998). Most studies to date have emphasized the burden and the negative psychological consequences of caregiving. It is only recently that attention has turned to the negative impact of caregiving on the physical health of the family caregiver.

Only a few studies have addressed the extent to which caregiving increases physical morbidity among caregivers. Morbidity indicators that have been explored or proposed include an increase in "minor" physical illness such as sleep disturbance and colds and an increased incidence of major physical illness such as hypertension, weight loss or gain, and anemia. Others have proposed that caregiving may be associated with under-, over-, and misuse of medications; drug and alcohol abuse; and troublesome symptoms such as poor appetite, smoking, exhaustion, and loss of energy.

Concern for family caregivers caring for relatives at the end of life

Health care professionals generally, and nurses specifically, have demonstrated an interest in promoting the physical and mental well-being of family caregivers providing palliative to a sick relative at the end of life. Hospice exemplifies a health care model that addresses the needs of family caregivers.

From hospice and other work in palliative care, two areas emerge as pivotal to nurses' role in improving and sustaining the physical and mental well-being of family caregivers. The first area addresses the role of nurses in aiding family members during the process of delivering palliative and end-of-life care. Through their interactions nurses and others on the hospice team empower family members to meet their caregiving obligations to their dying relative. The second area involves the role of nurses in helping family caregivers at the "moment of death."

When someone is ill, in pain, or in other ways unable to direct their own care, family members take on the responsibility of "speaking on behalf of the patient." Of primary importance for family members is the inherent pledge they make to the sick relative to direct the care in such a way that it is delivered in a manner consistent with the sick person's wishes and values.

Nurses, along with other members of the hospice or palliative care team, help family members articulate the care that their sick relative would want. Nurses then help family caregivers to the best of their ability to deliver that care, to take and to cede responsibility in such a way that is consistent with family understandings, and to explain when and why situations deviate from expectations.

Of prime importance is the nurse's role in helping family caregivers achieve a sense of closure about the care they have given a dying relative. Family caregivers who feel that they have fallen short in meeting their caregiving responsibility experience considerable mental anguish. They relive the experience, often long after the sick family member has died. They continue to examine in what way they fell short, how they could have improved on their behavior, and where and how they might have been more aggressive. There is an element of shame in not delivering on an implicit promise to the sick person. As such, the family member's recovery may be blocked. They may have somatic complaints or be unable to work to capacity or to enjoy life. We all know of family caregivers who relate over and over how a loved one died and how they, the responsible family member, was unable to control the environment, to make things happen (e.g., apply treatments, administer analgesics in a timely manner) in a way that is consistent with the values and expressed wishes of the sick family member. On the other hand, where family caregivers feel that they have been able to fulfill the promise to a loved on, they feel fulfilled, at peace, and accomplished in some way.

The second area in which nurses' involvement is critical to family caregivers is at the moment of death. Here nurses and others play a key role in bolstering a family member's strength in fulfilling their pledges to a family member (Mezey 2000). This is one of the crucial roles of hospice nurses, to come and be present at the moment of death. Family members often find it difficult to deliver on pledges when the patient is gasping for breath, flailing, or moaning. Here the nurses' role is to provide the memory and the strength for family members not to back down on their responsibility. Thus, in palliative and end-of-life care, professional responsibility extends directly to the family caregiver as "patient," positioning caregivers to regain their physical and mental health and empowering them to go on with their lives once their loved one has died.

Recommendations for Strengthening Nurses' Support of Family Caregivers

Adequate time for hospital and home care nurses to prepare family caregivers

Helping family members to take on caregiving tasks takes time. Mastery involves helping families practice and gain experience with tasks such as ambulation, dressing, bowel management, comfort care and pain management, dietary control, wound care, medication, and symptom management. Nurses voice concerns for family caregivers and a desire to help them acquire the needed skills to provide care. But nurses know that family members need time to acquire new information and to demonstrate their competency in providing care. In the hospital it is impressed upon the nursing, medical, and social work staff that "discharge planning begins on admission." In the current context of shortened stays, sicker patients, and fewer nurses, it is hard to imagine how hospital nurses can successfully prepare a patient for discharge, let alone adequately prepare a family member to provide the necessary care the patient will need when discharged. As one hospital nurse described it,: "This patient is post MI [myocardial infarction] and I (RN) have not had ten minutes to spend with him on patient education and he's going home today" (qtd. in Baer et al. 1996).

One of the assumptions of nurses working in hospitals is that, once the patient gets home, the home care nurse will have time to teach caregiving skills to the family. Yet, as noted, reimbursement for home care makes it increasingly unlikely that the professional home care nurse has time to teach and observe the caregiving skills of family members. Some models, such as that developed by Naylor et al. (1999), have shown the benefits that can accrue to both patients and family caregivers when the same nurse follows the patient in the hospital and at home. We will need to expand on this and other models if nurses are to carve out the time needed to prepare family members adequately for caregiving tasks.

Resolution of the current chaos in the home care industry

Between 1998 and 2000, 2,500 Medicare-certified home care agencies closed. Professional nurse staffing in home care has declined 23 percent since 1994. In some areas of the country patients are being discharged to long-term care facilities because home care is not available. New reporting requirements are substantially increasing the amount of time professional nurses in home care spend on paperwork. The new Outcome and Assessment Information Set (OASIS) questionnaire, required by Medicare to determine home care needs, is said to consume four hours of professional nurse time per patient (NYSNA report 2000). Thus, the core requirements for "doing business" are impeding home care nurses' ability to take on the added need to educate and support family caregivers.

A sense of stability will need to be reestablished before the home care industry can adequately take on responsibility for addressing the needs of family caregivers. Reimbursement changes proposed in the Medicare Prospective Payment system, with emphasis on clinical judgment as the basis for care, might provide a unique opportunity to focus on chronic illness and to strengthen the relationship between family caregivers and nurses in home care.

Linking home care agencies with academic nursing

Both patients and nurses in hospitals, and to a lesser extent long-term care facilities, have benefited from strong linkages with academic nursing programs. The experience of the Veterans Administration Hospitals with medical schools and the Robert Wood Johnson Foundation Teaching Nursing Home Program attest to the benefits of clinical agencies and academic setting jointly focusing on the clinical and research needs of patients and family members. Often such linkages result in the development of an agenda that capitalizes on the strengths of both institutions (Mitty and Mezey 1998; Naylor and Buhler-Wilkerson 1999).

Somewhat surprisingly, there are virtually no models of strong linkages between home care agencies and academic nursing programs (Mitty and Mezey 1998). Typically, nursing programs use home care agencies for episodic clinical experiences for baccalaureate or graduate nursing students. Creating more substantive linkages could strengthen a common commitment to addressing the needs of family caregivers, with a special focus on creating the curriculum and the science that would move such an agenda forward.

Conclusion

We continue to struggle with how much collective responsibility American society is willing to bear for the care of the chronically ill versus how much of the burden of care the individual and family must assume alone and without recourse (Lynaugh 1996). Family members today are assuming increasing responsibility for care of their sick relatives. Yet there is little evidence at the federal, state, or local level that bolstering family caregivers is a central agenda of health care.

Family caregivers and nurses share a historical reservoir of commitment to improve the ability of families to care for the sick. Traditionally, family members have turned to nurses to assist them in providing care to sick relatives at home. Family members continue to seek nurses' help, but all too often they find the response of nurses lacking in both substance and effort. Nurses, on the other hand, have a long-standing commitment to assist family caregivers. Clinical and academic nursing programs have a growing, albeit underdeveloped, agenda to support families. What is left to be seen is the extent to which family members and nurses can work together to create the regulatory and reimbursement climate needed to bolster family caregivers.

ACKNOWLEDGMENTS

The author gratefully acknowledges review of this chapter by Karen Buhler-Wilkerson and the research assistance of Abraham Brody in preparing it.

REFERENCES

Abt Associates, Inc. (2000, Apr. 13). "Evaluation of Community Nursing Organization Demonstration Projects: Final Report." Prepared for Health Care Financing Administration, Cambridge, Mass.

Arras J., and N. Dubler. (1994). "Bringing the Hospital Home: Ethical and Social Implications of High-Tech Home Care." *Hastings Center Report* 249(5):S19–28.

Baer, E., C. Fagin, and S. Gordon, eds. (1996). *The Abandonment of the Patient: The Impact of Profit-Driven Health Care on the Patient.* New York: Springer.

Branch, L. G., R. F. Coulam, and Y. A. Zimmerman. (1995). "The PACE Evaluation: Initial Findings." *Gerontologist* 35(3):349–59.

Buhler-Wilkerson K. (2001). *No Place like Home: A History of Nursing and Home Care in America.* Baltimore: Johns Hopkins University Press.

Buhler-Wilkerson, K., M. Naylor, S. Holt, and L. Rinke. (1998). "An Alliance for Academic Home Care: Integrating Research, Education, and Practice." *Nursing Outlook* 46:77–80.

Eleazer, G. P., et al. (1996). "Managed Care for the Frail Elderly: The PACE Project." *Journal of South Carolina Medical Association* 90:586–91.

Eng, C., J. Pedulla, P. Eleazer, R. McCann, and N. Fox. (1997). "Program of All-Inclusive Care for the Elderly (PACE): An Innovative Model of Integrated Geriatric Care and Financing." *Journal of the American Geriatric Society* 45:223–32.

Ferrell, B. (2001). "Pain Observed: The Experience of Pain from the Family Caregiver's Perspective." *Clinics in Geriatric Medicine* 7(3):595–609.

Given, B., and C. Given. (1998). "Health Promotion for Family Caregivers of Chronically Ill Elders," in Fitzpatrick J. J., ed. *Annual Review of Nursing Research,* 16:197–218. New York: Springer.

Health Care Financing Administration (HCFA). (2001). *National Health Expenditure Projections 2000–2010.* Washington, D.C.: Author.

Health Forum. (2000). *Hospital Statistics.* American Hospital Association. Chicago: Author.

Leff, B., and J. Burton. (2001). "The Future History of Home Care and Physician House Calls in the United States." *Journal of Gerontology: Biological Sciences and Medical Sciences* 56A:M603–M608.

Levine, C. (2000). *Rough Crossings.* New York: United Hospital Fund.

Lynaugh, J. (1996). "A Historical Perspective." In E. Baer, C. Fagin, and S. Gordon, eds., *The Abandonment of the Patient: The Impact of Profit-Driven Health Care on the Patient,* 73. New York: Springer.

Mezey, M. (2000, Sept. 13). "Comments on Family Caregiving," Conference on Palliative Care, Jewish Home and Hospital, New York.

Mitty, E., and M. Mezey. (1998). "Integrating Advanced Practice Nurses in Home Care: Recommendations for a Teaching Home Care Program." *Nursing and Health Care Perspectives* 19(6):264–70.

National Association of Home Care (NAHC). (2000, Mar). *Basic Statistics about Home Care.* Washington, D.C.: Author.

National Family Council Association (NFCA). (2000, Oct). *Caregiving Survey—2000.* Kensington, Md.: Author.

Naylor, M. D. (2000). "A Decade of Transitional Care Research with Vulnerable Elders." *Journal of Cardiovascular Nursing* 14(3):1–14.

Naylor MD., D. Brooten, R. Campbell, B. S. Jacobsen, M. D. Mezey, M. V. Pauly, and J. S. Schwartz. (1999). "Comprehensive Discharge Planning and Home Follow-up of Hospitalized Elders: A Randomized Clinical Trial." *JAMA* 281(7):613–20.

Naylor, M. D., and K. Buhler-Wilkerson. (1999). "Creating Community-based Care for the New." *Nursing Outlook* 47:120–27.

New York State Nurses Association (NYSNA). (2000, Feb.). *Report* (NYSNA newsletter).

Rinke, L., and S. Holt. (2000). "Primary Care in the Home: The Time Is Now!" *Home Health Care Management Practice* 12:1–9.

Schumacher, K. L., B. J. Stewart, P. G. Archbold, M. J. Dodd, and S. L. Dibble. (2000). "Family Caregiving Skill: Development of the Concept." *Research in Nursing and Health* 23(3):191–203.

Stewart, B. J., P. G. Archbold, K. S. Lyons, N. Perrin, T. Harvath, R. J. V. Montgomery, J. H. Carter, C. Waters, J. Lear, I. Inoue, J. Kaye, F. Miller, and T. Keane. (2001). "The Factor Structure of Caregiver Role Strain Is More Complex with More Strain." *Gerontologist* 41(Special Issue 1): 101–2.

Stone, R. (2001). "Putting Care Back into Home and Community Based Services." In *The Lost Art of Caring,* ed. R. Binstock and L. Cluff. Baltimore: Johns Hopkins University Press.

Vladeck, B. (2000). "The Storm before the Calm before the Storm: Medicare Home Care in the Wake of the Balanced Budget Act." *Case Management Journals* 2(4):232–37.

CHAPTER SIX

The Culture of Home Care

Whose Values Prevail?

Rick Surpin and Eileen Hanley

Care in the home is dramatically different from care in a hospital or nursing home. In a hospital the patient, albeit the focus of attention, may feel reduced to the object of the endless ministrations and questions of anonymous questioners. The family feels even more estranged, hovering around the patient or pursuing the staff for information or assistance.

In the home it is the professional and paraprofessional caregivers who are outsiders. They are "guests," although the patient or family may only have agreed to let them in, not invited them specifically. Because we usually think of a patient as a person lying in a hospital bed, wearing an unattractive gown that identifies his or her patienthood status, it even seems inappropriate to call someone a "patient" in his or her own home.

All the ways that institutions assert their control over patients and their families are absent in the home. The situation is reversed. Home is the patient's turf. Doctors, the chief representatives of the culture of medicine, rarely even enter the patient's home. Because of its context, home care is inherently an ongoing process of accommodation between the cultures of medicine and nursing (subcategory home care) and the culture of families. None of the people who are involved have sufficient power to control everything that happens. Because power in this case is embedded in relationships—patient, family, nurses, aides—it also shifts frequently.

This chapter will explore the particular ways in which cultural conflict arises in home care and the process of accommodation which attempts to resolve differences of worldview. We will pay particular attention to the front-line paid caregivers, the indispensable home care aides who in many ways are more like family caregivers than professionals but whose jobs are defined and actions governed by the culture of professionals and, significantly, of public policy. A brief historical detour may help illuminate how home care came to be defined, provided, and regulated and how this process established both the parameters of care and the potential for conflict.

Home Care: A Historical Perspective

Before the twentieth century almost all medical care was home care (see Chapter 4, by Sheila Rothman, in this volume). Only the destitute and abandoned were taken to hospitals or asylums, and even then it was mostly to die or languish. In the twentieth century, as scientific medicine began to take root, hospitals became the locations of choice for many types of care (see Chapter 5, by Mathy Mezey, in this volume). Although private-duty nurses in the first part of the century enjoyed a great deal of autonomy, their opportunities for employment were limited to families who could afford to pay them. They had limited contact with other health providers on the job and were often treated as domestic servants by their patients and families. Their work was also erratic and mostly obtained through private registries or doctors' recommendations. Since the private-duty nurse was neither family nor servant, there was no clear role for her in the daily life of the household. As nursing increasingly became hospital based and specialized, especially after World War II, it became separated from the sphere of domestic work.

Yet the role of providing personal care and assistance with household tasks for chronically ill patients and their families remained. Families themselves did most of the work. To the extent that paid caregivers were involved, they were mostly licensed practical nurses (LPNs), who had more limited education and training than registered nurses (RNs), and by home care aides for the small number of families who could afford to pay for such services or who received free or subsidized services from a public hospital or nonprofit visiting nurse service.

Visiting nurse services began as a charitable venture of the pre–Civil War women of Charleston, South Carolina, who combined prevailing ideals of religious duty and domestic skills to provide care to the poor (Buhler-Wilkerson 2001). Then, as now, the caregivers and patients were primarily women.

As home care developed in the early twentieth century, the visiting nurse's mission was "to care for the sick, to teach the family how to care for its sick family member, and to protect the public from the spread of disease through forceful yet tactful lessons in physical and moral hygiene" (Buhler-Wilkerson 2001, 204). The home care nurse was seen as a public health generalist who was responsible for a variety of medical, health, and social service problems in poor communities. The nurse's "client" was the entire community, and she often conducted classes in community centers in basic health and parenting skills as well as visiting the homes of the sick. She acted as a skilled professional as well as filling the role today held by paraprofessionals assisting with personal care and homemaking needs. The standards for home and public health nursing were those imposed by the profession itself and not by any regulatory body. Reimbursement for this service was either through philanthropic funds or based on the family's ability to pay.

As private-duty nursing gradually declined and hospital employment grew, public health nursing became the major way to provide care in the home. The context for home care and visiting nurse services changed dramatically, however, with the introduction of Medicare and Medicaid in 1965, which established the current framework in which much home care, and certainly all publicly funded home care, is provided.

The Creation of a New Job Description: The Home Care Aide

Medicare (a federal program for people over sixty-five and some disabled people) and Medicaid (a federal-state program for poor people) changed the home care field dramatically. These new programs provided much needed funding for home care services but also established new definitions of services and scope of practice. Federal and state regulations, not the nursing profession, defined the standards and practice of what constituted home care. The nursing role was narrowed to cover "homebound" patients recovering from an acute illness or trauma, rather than patients who needed mainly social and personal care support and rather than the community as a whole.

Home care was not a major consideration when Medicare and Medicaid were introduced. Home care services were seen as the medical needs that were left over after hospitalization. As A. E. Benjamin points out, "No theme in home care's recent history is stronger than its reliance for legitimacy on reducing the use and costs of inpatient acute and nursing-home care," even though there is ample evidence that home care does not necessarily reduce these costs (1993, 159). From the beginning policy makers worried that too much or too easy access to home care would encourage families to give up their unpaid caregiving. Despite many studies that show that family caregivers do not abandon their relatives when some formal care is provided, this theme constantly recurs in policy discussions.

Following the medical model, home care services were divided into "skilled and "unskilled." Skilled services include such activities as wound care, infusion therapies, and medication administration. Only trained and licensed nurses (and untrained family members) are legally allowed to provide these services. Unskilled services include personal hygiene, feeding, and meal preparation as well as some homemaking tasks. These are the domains of the home care aide. (There are various titles for this job, including personal care attendant, home health aide, and home care aide; there are technical distinctions among them, but, for simplicity, we will refer to these workers as home care aides.) Over time bodies of regulations were put in place to codify the division between skilled and unskilled services. The regulations place nurses in the dominant, supervisory position. Home care aides are subordinate and, by the very designation of providing unskilled labor, occupy a position something but not exactly like that of domestic workers. Their work, like that of family members, is considered unexceptional, like "housework" or, more likely, "women's work." Consistent with their origin as temporary employment agencies for hospitals and nursing homes, many agencies consider aides to be hourly workers with no benefits or job security. Nurses, however, are typically salaried and have comprehensive benefits.

The nurse frames the plan of care, taking on the role held by the physician in acute care (although physicians' orders are still required). The nurse's primary focus is on the patient, not on the aide or the family. Although nurses are technically the aides' supervisor, they have rarely been trained or directed in ways that would help them supervise and support the aides. Visits to the home are often made when aides are not there. The home care nurse has less time to devote to the needs of family caregivers and home care workers due to the increasing demands on his or her time and the unwillingness of payers to cover activities that are not directly performed for the patient.

The reimbursement streams have also defined new requirements for payment such as "part-time" and "intermittent" care. These distinctions were not based in home care practice but, rather, in assumptions and fears about the potentially unmanageable demand for and cost of home care services. (See Chapter 7, by Judith Feder and Carol Levine, in this volume.) Indeed, home care costs did rise precipitously in the late 1980s. This trend was mostly fueled by the emergence of a large number of small for-profit providers in the South and Southwest which emerged after the federal 1988 decision in *Duggan v. Bowen* loosened restrictions on the number of nursing/aide visits that could be made. The inevitable reaction resulted in the severe congressional cutbacks in the Balanced Budget Act of 1997. Although some of these cuts have been restored, the reimbursement requirements have continued to become more rigorous.

Recent reimbursement changes in Medicare force the nurse to change her focus from the patient to the specific medical problem, such as the body part or the wound. It is task oriented with a specific clinical outcome in mind. For home care aides changes in reimbursement have resulted in fewer hours of service per week with each patient and a more intense focus on tasks performed.

The nurse typically makes a visit for fifteen to thirty minutes. It is the home care aide who spends more time with the patient and family, although this, too, varies. On a typical Medicare case the aide may spend two to three hours a day for three to five days a week. Medicaid cases can range from two to twelve to twenty-four hours, three to five to seven days a week, depending on the specific regulations of the particular state and county.

Home care aides typically have minimal training, low pay, few if any benefits, and erratic, part-time work. They may be assigned several cases a day and are often not paid for travel time. Like other people who are working but poor, their personal lives are stitched together and can easily unravel. Lacking the clear boundaries of an institutional facility, these problems can easily spill over into patients' homes. Patients and family members who value a particular aide and do not want to see him or her leave may become enmeshed in trying to solve these often intractable problems, with money, advice, or advocacy. This is not a professional relationship nor a friendship but something in between; few people know intuitively how to be compassionate and kind and still set boundaries.

Of the 2.1 million paraprofessionals in the health care system, about 746,000 work in home care and the rest in nursing homes or hospitals as Certified Nursing Assistants (CNAs). The overwhelming majority (over 80 percent) are women. While most of them (55 percent) are white, there is a substantial minority component, with 35 percent black and 10 percent Hispanic. In urban centers with large immigrant populations, minority groups make up a greater percentage. Most aides work in agencies, although there is a substantial "gray market" in which aides work directly for patients and families through a registry or informal referral.

Home care aides are the lowest-paid workers in the health care system. Many work at minimum hourly wages ($5.15); at the higher end a worker might make about $11 or $12 an hour. The average national wage in 2003, according to the Bureau of Labor Statistics, was $8.46 an hour. (Registered nurses and professional therapists earn, on average, eighteen to twenty dollars per hour.) Aides working through agencies must follow the constraints of fairly extensive rules, from two main sources. First, Medicare and Medicaid regulations define allowable tasks. These definitions are meant to draw a line short of nursing tasks, which are generally defined in state nursing practice laws. Second, agencies establish operating procedures to set appropriate limits for what the aide can and cannot do.

These boundaries are rational attempts to make a distinction between family and paid caregivers. Yet family members with no training can do more tasks than aides are technically allowed to do. And agency procedures often set limits that are rational from the view of an office but not in the home— such as preparing meals for the patient but not for the spouse. At the same time, there must be limits on the homemaking aspect of the job; aides should not be asked to paint rooms or to wash windows. Finally, family members often need and expect more services, more hours, more relief, from their burden than the payer allows. From their viewpoint performing a variety of tasks and spending time with the patient to develop a relationship is exactly what is required. This is how people typically envision a caring experience in the home. They also think of the aide as an addition to the family—although often as their "girl" or their "maid."

These expectations are nearly the polar opposite of what Medicare and Medicaid expect to pay for. They are willing to pay for the time needed to perform specific tasks, not to build caring relationships. While local agencies deliver that message, it is the aide who must constantly negotiate private adjustments between the regulatory and economic constraints and the expectations and desires of patients and their families. The negotiations are often separate from the nurse and the agency. When they break down, it becomes a "silent war," until it is no longer tolerable for one of the combatants.

A Process of Accommodation between Cultures

Despite the barriers, many patients, families, nurses, and home care aides do manage to engage in a delicate process of negotiation, compromise, and accommodation (Collopy, Dubler, and Zuckerman 1990). This process includes recognition that family caregivers' lives have been significantly altered by the needs of their ill or infirm loved one. Their needs must be balanced with those of the beneficiary client. Family caregivers may be feeling anxious about their ability to render the necessary care correctly or their ability to handle any situation that may arise, or they may be feeling particularly conflicted between their sense of duty as a caregiver and the stress they feel as a result of their caregiver role.

To shape the process of accommodation and achieve better outcomes, the patient, as well as the formal and family caregivers, must constantly clarify a particular family's culture and how it relates to the professionals' and paraprofessionals' culture. Understanding a family's culture; knowing the style, values, and background of the home care provider; and examining the care plan itself all require effort and vigilance.

Family Culture
1. Is the client the patient or the family? Who constitutes the family? Is it a patient and one family member? Or are there several family members living in the home? Are the relationships based on birth, marriage, commitment, friendship? What role does each person play, and does this change over time?

2. Who are the decision makers in the family? Is the process of decision making collaborative or autocratic?

3. What are the inherent conflicts within the family? How, if at all, do these conflicts influence caregiving or the lack of it? Whose wishes take precedence, and what are those wishes? Is there coercion on the part of the patient, a family member, the professional, or the home care aide?

4. What is the class and ethnic background of the patient and family members? Are there generational, social, or economic differences that affect caregiving?

5. Is this a new event in the patient's and family's life? Family care-givers who have been through months and years of chronic illness are often experts at providing or supervising even complex medical care. They can explain how things should be done or how the patient reacts to particular procedures. When the experience is new, however, even ordinary tasks seem overwhelming. If a nurse or aide does not appear confident or questions prior instructions, the family and patient often become anxious or suspicious.

The Home Care Providers

6. Is a nurse involved? How often does she visit? With whom does she interact? What is her background, her ideas about family responsibility, her communication style?

7. Is a home care aide involved? How often is she there? With whom does she interact? What is her background, her ideas about family responsibility, her communication style?

8. Who is paying for the care? Is the family providing all of the care themselves? If so which ones? Is the family paying for formal care-giving on a private basis? If so, which family member(s)? What kind of agency is being used—for example, a registry, a licensed home care agency, a Medicare-certified agency? When the family pays, the patient or the dominant family member has more power in the relationship. When a third party is paying, usually Medicare or Medicaid, the regulations frame the relationship, and the nurse is more dominant. The aide is usually caught in the middle.

The Care Plan

9. Does the care require new equipment in the home such as a hospital

bed? Has it been ordered and provided, and is what is delivered what is really needed?

10. How medicalized is the care? Complex home care technology is a skilled service, and so a nurse will be involved. If the care requires use of high-tech equipment such as monitors and telemedicine, it will require a high level of attention from nurses, doctors, and/or technicians. The more the home looks and feels like a hospital, the more power in the relationship falls to the nurses, physicians, and technicians, and the more anxious the patient and family caregiver become. Some unskilled tasks, however, such as bathing a demented or paralyzed person, can be as or more difficult than a so-called skilled task, such as giving an injection.

The more complex the family situation and the care plan, the more complex the potential areas of conflict can be. One of the greatest areas of potential conflict occurs when care is not rendered according to someone's expectations. Perhaps the nurse believes that the family caregiver or paraprofessional is not adequately performing care. Perhaps the family caregiver believes that the paraprofessional is not performing according to his or her expectations. Clarifying and explaining each or these roles is the area that may require the most flexibility among all the parties and which must continue to be addressed over time.

Formal caregivers are often quick to label family caregivers or patients themselves as noncompliant rather than trying to find out the reasons behind the so-called noncompliance. In these situations the professional must become a detective to try to determine what is contributing to the problems and then determine a solution that does not compromise the care of the patient but which may be more acceptable to the family caregivers. It is important to determine whether the "noncompliance" is related to discomfort or pain;, lack of training, understanding, or commitment; or perhaps the financial resources needed to provide the expected care.

Friction can also occur when a particular treatment or procedure is uncomfortable for the patient. This can cause the family caregiver to become hesitant or stressed. Inflicting discomfort or pain or being on the receiving end of an angry outburst from the patient feels quite different to the professional who can rationalize that the treatment is beneficial to the patient and, therefore, not take the resistant behavior as personal criticism. This is not always the case when a family member is providing the care. The intimacy required for some of the care may also be a source of embarrassment for both the family member and the patient.

Over time the informal caregivers may become quite expert at rendering care that is skillful and comfortable for the client. They may be so attuned to the patients' needs that a new nurse on the case could have difficulty meeting the needs of the patient in the same way. The nurse may feel that he or she has the professional expertise to render the care correctly and does not wish to take direction from a nonprofessional family member or even the patient. At varying times the nurse can be seen as colleague, supervisor, teacher, caregiver, subordinate, or hired help. This shifting identity can be a barrier to effective caregiving by each party.

In addition to the conflicts that home care nurses may feel with patients and/or their family, they may be experiencing internal conflicts as well. This occurs most often when a nurse feels conflicted between his or her role as advocate and gatekeeper. Many nurses would prefer never to have to discuss with patients or families the fact that their insurance will not pay for a certain piece of equipment or that the nurse's visits and those of the home care aide will be discontinued abruptly. Yet this is a constant part of the job, and it often causes much stress for the home care professional.

Policy Implications

The current fee-for-service Medicare and Medicaid long-term care system has dramatically narrowed the boundaries in which the process of accommodation among patient, family, nurses, and aides takes place. Both public and private payers of home care operate on the basis of "this is what we are willing to pay for" and not "this is what we will do in collaboration with you." Family care is the predominant form of assistance to elderly and disabled people requiring care in their homes. It should be interwoven with the formal care system—not treated as a separate system that must be essentially depleted before formal services are called upon. Furthermore, the formal system must become more flexible and able to respond to a client's changing needs. Even though a long-term client has a "chronic condition," that condition can change instantly—a broken hip, heart failure, the death of a spouse—and the system of care must adapt just as quickly.

At the same time, the formal system is facing a deepening crisis as both nurses and home care aides are in increasingly short supply. Nurses are leaving the profession primarily due to onerous paperwork requirements, and enrollments in nursing school have continued to decline. It has become significantly harder to attract potential workers to become home care aides when the jobs do not offer full-time employment, a livable wage, family health benefits, adequate training, or supportive working conditions. This situation will only worsen as the elderly population increases and the pool of available workers decreases over the next twenty to thirty years.

The combination of the stresses on the family caregiving system and the growing shortage of nurses and home care aides will require developing a new model for long-term care based on collaboration between and among family caregivers and formal caregivers. Such a model will require a fundamental restructuring of our long-term care system, and it will not happen soon. There are, however, experiments across the country seeking to address some of the basic issues discussed here. We believe that the experiments with the most potential for long-term impact are programs seeking to coordinate services for long-term care clients across the various care settings, to integrate medical and social needs, and to blend formal caregiving with family and volunteer caregiving. The Programs of All-Inclusive Care for the Elderly (PACE) On Lok programs and the Community Medical Alliance in Massachusetts are the early forerunners of this design. New models are also emerging using a broader community setting, including VNS Choice, a managed long-term program for the elderly in New York City sponsored by the Visiting Nurse Service of New York; the Wisconsin Partnership Program; and our own Independence Care System (ICS), a managed long-term care program for adults with physical disabilities in New York City sponsored by the Paraprofessional Healthcare Institute and Cooperative Home Care Associates.

These programs have in common a comprehensive framework and a focus on interdisciplinary care management and coordination of services. They broaden the framework beyond care at home to both the full range of home- and community-based services and to the relationship with primary and acute medical care providers. The emphasis on care management gives these programs greater capacity to address problems as they arise and to involve other service providers in the process. At the same time, they are faced with constantly trying to adjust their "mental models" of the way the long-term care system should work to the organizational and fiscal realities of the current system.

One of the areas in which these programs differ from more traditional long-term care is in their focus on the consumer as not just the center of the plan but in fact the director of the plan. At ICS the philosophy of care coordination and management emphasizes that the consumer has the right and responsibility to direct his or her own care. This is a significant departure from the more traditional and paternalistic attitude of many health care entities that the professional and formal caregivers "know best." At ICS much time is spent working with care managers, other staff members, and contracted paraprofessional agencies to learn how best to help members become more self-directing and how to work with those who are already functioning somewhat autonomously. It does not always come easily for members or staff. Orientation and training helps staff to focus on their members' strengths and abilities rather than on what they cannot do. Focusing on long-term goals and desires and the need for intermediate steps to meet these goals is an important aspect of the development of staff as well as the member. Training programs are often conducted by people living with disabilities themselves who not only can articulate issues from a perspective of a member but also can serve as role models for members who may be feeling intimidated at the thought of gaining more autonomy.

The ICS philosophy carries over to the paraprofessional agencies that work with ICS clients. It is made clear to agencies that ICS is approaching care management in a different way and that the role of the home care worker is expected to be less traditional than usual. ICS expects the home care workers to be equal and contributing members of the care management team. This often requires skills development in communication techniques, problem solving, and assessment. The paraprofessional needs to learn to negotiate an environment in which the client may be very self-directing and the worker may be worried about safety, for instance, or issues that may arise from conflicts in lifestyle decisions. Family members when involved as caregivers are also involved in decision making about care management. This shift in approach will continue to evolve and require a different type of training for all involved.

These programs will especially generate pressure to respond to needs that are not addressed in the fee-for-service Medicare and Medicaid system—for example, wheelchair maintenance and minor repair, maintenance physical therapy (not only restorative), and informal social centers. There will be corresponding pressure to contain the overall cost of services and treat anything new as a substitute for something currently provided. This, too, is a process of ongoing accommodation—of push and pull—and we hope that, as the experiments mature, they will provide the foundation for a truly new system of long-term care.

These experiments will be evaluated by a variety of different criteria over the next decade especially regarding cost effectiveness. Yet an equally important test that must not be lost as we seek to restructure the system that we have today is: Do the new models recognize and effectively support the continuous balancing act between patient, family, nurses, and aides in the home? Our hope and belief is that we will be able to say yes to this question as the experiments mature. Participants and observers alike should recognize, however, that there are key tests to pass before anybody can say that we have a new model that works.

REFERENCES

Benjamin, A. E. (1993). "An Historical Perspective on Home Care Policy." *Milbank Quarterly* 71(1):129–66.

Buhler-Wilkerson, K. (2001). *No Place like Home: A History of Nursing and Home Care in the United States.* Baltimore: Johns Hopkins University Press.

Collopy, B., N. N. Dubler, and C. Zuckerman. (1990, Mar.–Apr.). "The Ethics of Home Care: Autonomy and Accommodation." *Hastings Center Report.*

Paraprofessional Healthcare Institute. (2001, Jan.). "Direct-Care Health Workers: The Unnecessary Crisis in Long-Term Care." Report. New York.

Stone, R. L., with J. M. Wiener. (2001, Oct.). *Who Will Care for Us? Addressing the Long-Term Care Workforce Crisis.* Washington, D.C.: Urban Institute and Institute for the Future of Aging Services.

Part III / The Societal Context

CHAPTER SEVEN

Explaining the Paradox of Long-Term Care Policy

An Example of Dissonant Cultures

Judith Feder and Carol Levine

Who creates all the rules and regulations that bedevil (even as they benefit) family caregivers? Health policy makers. The category may sound abstract, but it describes real people who shape the ways medical care and social services are delivered, paid for, and regulated. Health policy makers include elected officials, such as members of Congress, state legislators, governors, and the president; appointed officials, such as the administrator of the Center for Medicare and Medicaid Services (CMS, formerly the Health Care Financing Administration) and state Medicaid directors; the political appointees and civil servants who work for all these sectors; and managers in private organizations that contract with government agencies to administer public programs. Like the health care professionals described in other chapters in this book, health policy makers also have a particular culture that governs their attitudes, assumptions, and values.

This chapter aims to shed light on the culture clash between policy makers and family caregivers by exploring the factors that underlie a major area of controversy—Medicare policy toward care at home. A fundamental assumption underlying health care policy, whether public or private, is that the legal beneficiary is an individual, not a family. Even a family member covered by the same program as an individual or a dependent is still considered a separate beneficiary. Family caregivers as family caregivers are not entitled to anything beyond what they might receive as individual beneficiaries. Furthermore, while policy makers are concerned about promoting access to quality care, they tend to view programs as they affect the full population they are intended to serve, rather than programs' impacts on particular individuals. Their focus is on the benefits the law provides to program beneficiaries, not on the varied circumstances facing beneficiaries and their families. And their actions reflect their responsibility to balance the legal and fiscal integrity of programs with beneficiaries' access to care. In short, their perspective is very different from that of family caregivers, who are concerned with the needs and preferences of individuals in the context of the family. And the very actions that, viewed from the policy makers' perspective, seem essential to responsible program administration may be seen by caregivers as illogical or even perverse barriers to achieving the best and most comprehensive care for their ill relatives.

Given these basic assumptions and values, it is not surprising that specific rules and regulations often baffle beneficiaries and their family caregivers. In this chapter we address a series of questions that caregivers often ask: Why doesn't Medicare cover long-term care? Why is the limited coverage Medicare home health provides seemingly so arbitrary or illogical? Why do providers so often say, "Medicare (or any other insurance) won't pay"? And why do home health coverage rules seem at odds with, rather than supportive of, caregiver needs? The purpose of this chapter is not to justify or vilify current policy and its limitations. Rather, it is to make policy more understandable and thereby provide some guidance to making it better.

Why Doesn't Medicare Cover Long-Term Care?

Many people who are eligible for Medicare—as well as their family caregivers—are surprised and dismayed to discover the limits to its benefits when they need long-term care. Indeed, the limits and barriers to Medicare home health benefits may be among the least comprehensible of the many financing frustrations that caregivers face. People in need of long-term care have a range of service requirements. Some, like housekeeping and grocery shopping, require little specialized skills or training; others, like medication management and physical therapy, require professional-level expertise. Beneficiaries and their family caregivers care more about getting appropriate services than about the differences among them. In trying to obtain Medicare home health benefits, beneficiaries and caregivers are often frustrated by rules that, from the family-centered culture, seem aimed at preventing them from getting the very benefits they believe the program was intended to provide.

From a policy perspective a fundamental distinction between skilled and unskilled services sets the parameters. In order for a beneficiary to receive Medicare benefits for unskilled services, such as those provided by an aide, Medicare rules require that he or she be determined to need skilled services, for example, those provided by a nurse. While these distinctions are clear to policy makers, they may make no sense at all to family caregivers, who view the care recipient's needs in their totality. Some of the tasks that are classified as skilled, such as giving an injection, may seem much less taxing than the unskilled job of bathing a demented or paralyzed patient. Although the full set of supports is essential to a person with impairments, Medicare is far more likely to cover the services that require professionally provided or medically related care than it is to cover unskilled support.

This differential treatment characterizes private as well as public insurance. But it is probably most disappointing when it arises within a public program—specifically, Medicare. The reasons for this differential treatment are neither ignorance nor meanness.

In fact, Medicare's statute, enacted in 1965, explicitly prohibits coverage of what is termed "custodial care." Although Medicare pays for some limited nursing home and home health care, the program's coverage policies reflect its focus on care needs directly associated with episodes of acute illness. It is Medicaid, a federal/state means-tested program—not Medicare—which is the nation's primary public support for people who need long-term care. Even when Medicare home health coverage policies were at their most expansive, in the early 1990s, only about 10 percent of elderly beneficiaries living at home who had impairments in activities of daily living were actually receiving Medicare home health benefits.

Medicare's statutory and operational limitations reflect a general aversion to insuring custodial or personal care which is almost as strong in the policy culture today as it was in 1965. Policy makers are concerned that, if insurance eliminates or substantially reduces the costs of service, people will use much more of it. And they believe more people will use it who did not do so before.

Making appropriate services available by reducing financial barriers is, of course, part of the purpose of insurance. But, if the potential increase in use is perceived as poorly tied to any measurable concept of need and administratively difficult to manage, then policy makers fear that costs will become uncontrollable. If that happens, the program will be unaffordable and unacceptable to the taxpayers who must support it.

Doesn't the risk that insurance will increase service use exist with acute care insurance? Of course it does. And, indeed, concerns about the program costs that will come with the aging of the baby boom generation have led some policy makers to question whether it is possible to continue to bear the risks of medical care through Medicare. But, that said, there is a greater reluctance to bear the risks associated with long-term care than there is for medical care. That's partly because of a belief that long-term care is a family responsibility, an issue that will be addressed later in this chapter. But it's also because of differences between medical and long-term care. In medical care policy makers can look to professional medical standards that, at least in theory, determine who gets what service. By contrast, in long-term care, much of the care is supportive and social in nature, and the links to and relationships between overall health status and functioning are not always clear or well understood. The benefit may have less to do with health status than with improving quality of life, a goal that is less measurable and perhaps less politically acceptable. Further, much medical care is invasive and unpleasant or painful to those who receive it. By contrast, help with household chores (if not always help with more hands-on services) is painless and may be welcomed as a relief to family caregivers.

Concern about the health care system's ability to control the costs of existing public programs for health care and reluctance to take on new responsibilities may lead policy makers to overstate the degree of financial risk that insurance coverage for long-term care would actually pose. Experience with Medicaid and with the newly emerging private long-term care insurance reveals that we do have the capacity to measure "need" and to distinguish people with significant impairments from the general population (elderly or otherwise). That experience indicates that policy measures can be used to target resources to people with the greatest need and to set limits on the scope of services provided. And patients' and families' reluctance to have a "stranger in the house" and many family caregivers' determination to "do it myself" may limit the extent to which family caregivers rely on formal services, even when they are made available.

Nevertheless, program management has operational and political costs. Operating a program means denying service to some who would like to receive it; limiting service to those who would like more service than the program is willing to provide; and committing to expenditures that, while perhaps not uncontrollable, are certainly not easy to control. Overall, then, the insurance protection that the caregiver culture views as an investment in financial relief and service support essential to quality of life is viewed in the policy and political culture as a fiscally and politically risky course of action which they might be foolish to undertake.

Why Do Public Coverage Rules Seem Arbitrary and Illogical?

Given the basic assumptions and values underlying health care policy, it is not surprising that the result is often specific rules and regulations that trouble beneficiaries and family caregivers. For example, the requirement that the Medicare recipient must be "homebound" to receive home health services may discourage caregivers from providing their ill family members the very activities that improve their quality of life. The definition of *homebound* is "normally unable to leave home." That is, the homebound care recipient can leave home only infrequently, for a short time, or to get medical care or attend religious services (the latter added in 2000 because of public pressure on Congress). The requirement exists because Congress wanted to provide skilled service benefits at home only to people who could not go out to receive them, say, to a clinic or rehabilitation facility—a strategy aimed at limiting Medicare's expenses. But the effect is to keep people at home when they might be able to enjoy a family outing, a museum visit, or another nonreligious activity. Financial intermediaries interpret the guidelines differently, and so caregivers who try to get patients "out of the house" to improve their spirits therefore may do so surreptitiously so as not to risk losing Medicare coverage.

The rules on coverage for durable medical equipment are difficult to interpret. Many Medicare recipients need some form of durable medical equipment—wheelchair, hospital bed, or other equipment. The proper wheelchair is essential for the recipient's mobility and prevention of muscle, joint, or skin problems. Yet Medicare will typically pay only for generic equipment that is "medically necessary," as certified by the physician—a criterion that often falls short of meeting a patient's full needs or preferences.

Similarly frustrating is Medicare's rule that limits coverage for rehabilitation services to patients who are making "progress." Clearly, even sustaining a level of functioning—that is, preventing deterioration—may require rehabilitation services. Why, then, wouldn't they qualify as covered services? The answer again has to do with the limited scope of Medicare coverage as the law defines it. Here, again, Medicare benefits, intended to be narrow from the start, are restricted to skilled services; so-called maintenance therapy can be performed by nontherapists and even family members—though family members may be unable or unwilling to do so.

In general, the barriers caregivers face reflect the policy culture's efforts to balance the desire to provide benefits with the desire to keep expenditures under control. The balance is unfortunately difficult to achieve and sometimes leads to policies that, viewed from the caregiver culture, seem totally irrational. Viewed from the caregiver culture, which emphasizes the specific circumstances of the affected family, it is hard to understand why a program would resist spending a modest amount on services at home, when that investment could prevent the far greater expense associated with a hospital stay or admission to a nursing home. From the policy perspective, however, paying for care at home poses some risks. One is that services formerly provided by unpaid family members will be transferred to the public sector, resulting in increased costs. This belief persists despite numerous studies showing that family members continue to provide substantial amounts of needed care even when public services are available. Another concern is that newly supported services at home would be in addition to, not just a replacement for, hospital or nursing home care. In some cases greater availability of home care would indeed prevent the use of more expensive hospital or nursing home services. But in others greater availability of home care would mean that some beneficiaries and families would use this benefit even if they had not considered using the hospital or nursing home.

Indeed, experience with Medicaid suggests that, unless there is aggressive financial control, when home health services are made more widely available, the costs associated with more people using service exceed the savings associated with reductions in hospital or nursing home care by some individuals. Program structure that seems arbitrary and illogical from the caregiver culture is therefore understandable in the policy culture as a rational mechanism for controlling costs.

Why Do Health Care Providers Claim That "Medicare Won't Pay?"

Sometimes, as noted earlier, Medicare really does not cover a specific service. Sometimes patients and caregivers are confused about the difference between Medicare and Medicaid and may believe that Medicare is covering something for another patient when in fact it is not. Sorting out what the "government" provides is a challenge for many beneficiaries and their caregivers.

This challenge is made even more problematic by variations in coverage from place to place. Inconsistencies arise, first, because intermediaries between Medicare—the payer—and the care recipient actually determine what claims get paid. CMS contracts with several private administrative agencies around the country to review claims. Although they are all subject to the same basic rules, in practice these agencies may have different standards for approving or denying particular kinds of claims. People who invest the time and energy in appealing denials often succeed in obtaining coverage; however, many people are either unaware of the appeal process or are too overwhelmed to apply. Consistency is a goal, but achieving it requires a dedication of time, effort, and resources from Medicare's central office which has been difficult to achieve.

Second, the actual delivery of services reflects totally independent decisions by private providers—in particular, Medicare-certified home health agencies. Although Medicare is a public program, the program buys services from private professionals and professional organizations. Limited by the conditions of participation, these practitioners nevertheless have considerable flexibility in deciding what services they are willing to provide and which people they are willing to serve—decisions that are influenced by the coverage rules and financial incentives the program creates. The incentives regarding home health coverage have varied considerably over time and in the last two decades have gone from restrictive to expansive to restrictive. It is the interplay among core rules, intermediary interpretation, and provider behavior which drives benefits.

In the early 1980s interpretation of coverage rules, like those described here, became very restrictive in an effort to limit Medicare spending. In the late 1980s challenges in the courts forced an easing of restrictions. In response, agencies became far more willing to provide services, and expenditures on home health care grew dramatically. Congress responded to the spending increase, not primarily by changing the coverage rules but by changing the manner in which home health agencies were paid. Until 1997 home health agencies were paid on a "cost" basis, giving them little incentive to be efficient or to limit the services they provided. In the Balanced Budget Act of 1997, however, Congress began introducing a new payment system—modeled on the hospital payment system developed in the 1980s—which sets payment in advance.

The move to "prospective payment" aims at promoting efficiency by creating incentives for agencies not to provide "too much" care. But, under a prospective payment system, unlike the previous cost-based system, providers are rewarded financially for providing less service, regardless of patient needs. Provider payment rates are fixed and largely independent of what providers spend. The less they spend, the more they retain. Even if the system is designed to pay more for sicker than for less sick patients, within any rate class agencies benefit financially from serving less sick patients, who require relatively little service, and from avoiding or providing less care to patients with extensive needs. Although the goal behind prospective payment is to promote efficiency, in the absence of clear service norms, the impact may simply be less care.

Why Do Program Structures Seem Unsupportive of Caregiver Needs?

The cultural dissonance between caregivers and policy makers goes well beyond access to particular kinds of service. At its most fundamental it reflects a difference in attitudes toward the role of informal versus formal caregivers in providing long-term care. Informal caregivers—family members and friends—are the primary source of long-term care in the nation, providing all the long-term care received by about three-quarters of elderly long-term care users in the community.

The importance of the informal caregiver role would probably not surprise most caregivers. They would likely see it as, first and foremost, a reflection of their commitment to their loved ones. But they would likely also see it as a reflection of the difficulty they have in finding, managing, and paying for reliable, affordable paid helpers to share in the enormous range of caregiving responsibilities. Viewed from the culture of caregiving, public policy to make affordable and competent home care assistance more readily available would not lead them to give up their caregiving. Rather, it would enable them to make fewer sacrifices in employment and quality of life and would supplement the considerable care they would continue to provide. In other words, it would constitute a public investment that reduces the costs that caregivers face and increases the value of overall care.

In the policy culture, by contrast, the "costs" of unpaid caregiving tend not to count. And the benefits, in terms of improved quality of life for impaired individuals and their families, are given a low priority. Instead, support for paid caregiving that in any way replaces or might replace unpaid caregiving is seen as a costly and largely unnecessary publicly financed substitute for care that family members are willing to provide.

Treatment of family caregiving as free labor is not unique to long-term care. Changes in the health care system which have shortened stays in hospitals, for example, have relied on family members to provide care that used to be provided by hospital staff. The result is reduced hospital expenses but increased family burdens. From society's perspective it is not clear that the result is negative; in other words, it might be an acceptable tradeoff in the public's view. It is also not clear, however, that the public understands that there is indeed such a tradeoff.

In long-term care it is the benefits of reducing family burdens which are given short shrift. Indeed, the policy culture seems to view caregiving for impaired family members as a responsibility that families not only must but ought to cope with, with minimal, if any, public support. As long as the policy culture's basic presumption is that family responsibility is open-ended and unlimited, policy is likely to regard support for caregivers as an unwise rather than a prudent investment.

Conclusion

As we approach the aging of the baby boom generation, the policy culture has begun what is bound to be a long and intense debate about government's role in spreading risk. Proposals to privatize social security and Medicare challenge government responsibility for spreading the risks of aging and illness through government-guaranteed and government-provided benefits. Under the privatizing proposals individuals would seek protection against risks through the marketplace—a marketplace that we know from experience tends to segment the better-off from the less well-off and the healthy from the sick. As a result, the relatively disadvantaged will be more, not less, dependent on themselves and their caregivers for financial and service support. And the distance between the policy culture and the caregiver culture will grow, not diminish.

The fundamental questions that must be raised to bring the policy and caregiver cultures together is: Are we as a society willing to share the burdens of caregiving? Is it the job of family members to bear full responsibility for their own? Or is the job of society to "insure" family members as well as people with impairments against the burdens associated with long-term care? And, if we are willing to spread the risk, how will we balance families' need for support against taxpayers' concern with expenditures?

The answers to these questions are not simple. But there will be no satisfactory answer until we raise the questions more directly and more often.

CHAPTER EIGHT

Family Caregivers in Popular Culture

Images and Reality in the Movies

Carol Levine and Alexis Kuerbis

Images shape perceptions. Whether images are created by written or spoken words, photographs, or film, they profoundly affect the emotions and expectations attached to everything from the food we buy to the wars we wage. We "imagine" how the world works and our place in it. In the twentieth century and beyond, one of the most powerful mediums for communication has undoubtedly been film. Movies or films on videotape provide entertainment, fun, thrills, and enlightenment. Films show us as we would like to be or as we hope to avoid becoming, and only rarely as we really are. As Norman Denzin, a sociologist with a particular interest in film, points out, "[By 1930] American society became a cinematic culture, a culture which came to know itself, collectively and individually, through the images and stories that Hollywood produced" (1995, 24).

With this power film shapes society's perceptions of the behaviors and attitudes that are considered admirable, acceptable, or abominable. Most filmmakers see themselves as artists responding to their own vision or as commercial producers gauging the public's mood. Few explicitly express a particular, much less a moral, viewpoint. Nonetheless, even in the most trivial ways films convey moral points of view about characters, plot development, and denouement. With or without intending to, films make judgments about people and the way they live and die.

How, then, do films present family caregiving? What are the images that both arise from and shape societal views about caregiving? This chapter surveys caregiving in films, setting aside the more specific use of video as an instructional tool and documentaries as portrayals of reality.* Illness creates drama, and drama shows how characters respond to conflict and crisis. How caregivers are presented in films affects not only society's expectations but also health care professionals' views of caregivers (they go to movies too) and how caregivers view themselves. Furthermore, these images are a powerful but unexamined force in shaping policy makers' views of family caregivers and their needs, challenges, and capabilities. Although some medical themes have been explored in the enormous literature on film, for example, Denzin's work (1991) on alcoholism in the movies and Peter Dan's account (2000) of doctors in the movies, no comparable study has been made of family caregiving in films.

In the 1930s and 1940s films in which rich people were ill usually included the generic character of "the nurse," a woman in a starched white uniform and cap who responded to the patient's and family's calls for help. She seemed to be on duty all the time. These are also films in which doctors made house calls, sometimes more than once a day. In the same period films portraying poor people who were ill, whether on the frontier or in urban slums, included the generic character of the "mother" or "wife," dispensing broth and sympathy. She, too, was always available. A doctor might be called, but usually he was too far away to reach the patient in time. Sometimes a family would not call a doctor or would make a tremendous sacrifice to do so because they did not have the money to pay him or goods to barter. While a study of those early images of caregiving would be instructive, for our purposes we will focus on more recent movies.

*Both are important and interesting subjects, as devoid in different ways of the life experiences of caregivers as are popular films. In brief, instructional videos, although they can be helpful, present the tasks of caregiving in a carefully controlled environment. The "care recipient" is usually a compliant, healthy stand-in. The narrator reads the how-to script in a reassuring voice. Documentaries, although more realistic, are selective. They are edited to present a particular point of view, often with large gaps in events and time. There are, to be sure, some excellent documentaries, including *Complaints of a Dutiful Daughter*, a 1995 film by Deborah Hoffman about her mother's Alzheimer disease.

Within this overall category we have identified five broad types: the invisible caregiver, the Gothic caregiver, the saintly caregiver, the eroticized caregiver, and the more-or-less realistic caregiver. Although there are many films that fit each of these categories, and some that fit more than one, we have selected those that seem most appropriate for each of the categories. This is an impressionistic, not a comprehensive, survey. And we have limited our attention to physical, not mental, illnesses, with the exception of a few references to films about Alzheimer disease, which figures so prominently in contemporary caregiver experience.

The Invisible Caregiver

Illness, particularly terminal illness, is a common theme in popular movies. Many of the portrayals of illness present the patient's perspective, in which he or she apparently struggles through the ordeal without a hands-on caregiver or with one who appears only peripherally. The protagonist may fall ill or become disabled and has to cope with new limitations. In many of these movies, however, no matter how debilitated the patient is, the more mundane and sometimes nasty parts of caregiving are limited or altogether absent.

We refer to these films as having an invisible caregiver because in these scenarios all of the caregiving work, such as giving medications, ordering supplies, dealing with insurance companies, doing housework, preparing meals, and helping to bathe and dress an ill individual, is accomplished without a trace of another helping hand. Even when there is someone present who the audience assumes is the primary caregiver, such as a spouse, this person is able to sit calmly at the bedside of the ill individual and deal solely with the emotional issues of the crisis.

The Doctor (1991), *Man on the Moon* (1999), and *Isn't She Great?* (2000) are three examples of this genre. Each of them follows the trials and tribulations of the main character, who suffers from cancer, the perennial disease of choice for film. In each case their loved ones, who seem to be extremely dedicated to their sick partners, are never shown doing any actual caregiving tasks. The patient sits serenely watching the ocean or lies in bed while friends visit. The messy side of the ordeal is ignored. In these movies caregiving is not glorified or overemphasized; it is completely absent.

In the biographical story of comedian Andy Kaufman, *Man on the Moon*, Kaufman, played by Jim Carrey, is diagnosed with advanced lung cancer, from which he eventually dies. In a scene prior to his death, a close friend of Kaufman's, Bob Zmuda, played by Danny DeVito, comes to visit Kaufman, who has been ravaged by chemotherapy. Kaufman sits on a lounge chair, covered in a blanket, facing the ocean, as Zmuda sits and talks with him. The scene is calm, peaceful, and reassuring. Even though the movie is based on a true story, Kaufman does not cough once through the entire scene, nor does he have any pressing physical needs. His girlfriend, the primary caregiver, is nowhere in sight. We are left to believe that Kaufman's illness is painless and has allowed time for peaceful reflection and a reconnecting with nature. This scene is representative of the manner in which Kaufman's illness is handled throughout the last half of the movie. Although he has a disease that seriously weakens his ability to breathe, the progression of the illness is reflected only through Carrey's makeup. Kaufman's eventual death seems to have been preceded by cosmetic changes, not bodily debilitation.

Apart from the cancer films, *On Golden Pond* (1981) is probably the most well-known film of this genre. Certainly, its star cast and the real-life relationship of Henry and Jane Fonda add to its luster. Henry Fonda plays an aging professor, Norman, who must confront his increasing memory problems, aided by his devoted wife, Ethel, played by Katharine Hepburn. Their daughter, Chelsea, played by Jane Fonda, arrives at their summer house on Golden Pond and begins to repair the years of distance from her emotionally cold father. The major scene in which Norman goes to pick strawberries and forgets his way back to the house, after having taken the same path for years, is compelling. On the whole, however, the film presents dealing with dementia and aging rather simplistically. In one of the final scenes Norman has what appears to be a heart attack. Ethel is distraught, and, in an attempt to will him to get better with her loving devotion, she cries that she loves Norman too much for him to die. Although the incident is frightening and emotional for the couple, Ethel's powers work their magic. The pains subside, and Norman is healthy after all. The end of the movie is only the beginning of Norman's decline, which we are led to believe will be as serene as Golden Pond itself.

The Gothic Caregiver

In this genre of caregiver portrayals, not only do caregivers exist; they are also cruel and sadistic. These "caregivers" in fact abuse the ill, rendering them helpless and dependent. The classic movies *Jane Eyre* (based on the Charlotte Brontë novel) and *Gaslight* are predecessors of this theme. In *Jane Eyre* Rochester locks his mad wife in an attic, and in *Gaslight* the husband attempts to drive his wife mad.

In movies such as *Misery* (1990) and *The Sixth Sense* (1999) the "care" of the patient is ironically complex and often difficult. Yet the caregiver also deviously plots both in secret and overtly to keep the patient immobilized, incapacitated, and within her total control. In these scenarios the patient is a victim, the caregiver a perpetrator.

In *Misery*, based on the novel by Stephen King, Kathy Bates plays Annie Wilkes, the "number one fan" of novelist Paul Sheldon, played by James Caan. After being severely injured in a car accident while stranded in a blizzard in the mountains, Wilkes becomes his accidental caregiver and slowly nurses him back to health. When Wilkes discovers that Sheldon has killed her favorite character in his latest book, she brutally handicaps her injured "patient" so that he is trapped in her house long enough to rewrite the publication. Wilkes takes great care to keep Sheldon healthy enough to write but resorts to such cruel tactics as breaking his ankles with a sledgehammer, crippling him permanently. King's novel and the movie make explicit a common but unspoken fear that illness and disability will render us helpless to the predatory motives of others.

In *The Sixth Sense* the victim is not as lucky, if that is the right word, as Sheldon. One of the ghosts haunting the clairvoyant, eleven-year-old Cole, played by Haley Joel Osment, is a young girl who has recently died after a long illness. Directed by the girl's ghost, Cole silently and painstakingly brings a video to the girl's father at a gathering after the funeral. The video reveals that the mother, while apparently vigilantly caring for their daughter, had slowly and methodically poisoned her with rat poison. Unlike *Misery*, the motive for such sadistic behavior is unclear. We are left to speculate. Was it Munchausen syndrome by proxy, a disorder in which a parent seeks attention and praise while actually orchestrating her child's illness and death? Was it a selfish scheme to be the sole recipient of her husband's attention? Like *Misery*, this sequence plays to an unconscious fear that the person on whom we are most dependent for care (Mother!) might betray us.

Another type of grotesque caregiver portrayal can be found in some films, loosely categorized as black comedy, depicting patients with Alzheimer disease or dementia. In films such as *Where's Poppa?* (1970) greedy family caregivers try to get control of the older person's fortune. In movies such as *Folks* (1992) bizarre behavior, memory loss, and inappropriate language are presented as humor. While these films may indeed be funny, they are gross distortions of what caregivers actually endure. There seems to be no middle ground between benign portrayals of the disease and tasteless exploitation. Realistic portrayals, especially in terms of the hostility, paranoia, and erratic behavior often manifested by people with Alzheimer's, are rare, perhaps non-existent.

The Saintly Caregiver

At the other extreme is the saintly caregiver, who goes beyond any expected reaction to illness and becomes a superhuman advocate and nurse. No task is too hard for the saintly caregiver, no prognosis too dire. This caregiver is more devoted, more knowledgeable, more passionate, than any professional or other family member. She never gives up.

Lorenzo's Oil (1992), based (loosely and apparently somewhat inaccurately) on a true story, presents one such caregiver team. Young Lorenzo Odone, played in the film by Zack O'Malley Greenburg, was diagnosed at the age of five with adrenoleukodystrophy (ALD), a disease characterized by the breakdown of the myelin sheath surrounding nerve cells in the brain. It leads to progressive dysfunction of the adrenal gland, which eventually leaves the victim helpless and unable to communicate.

Faced with this tragic prognosis, Lorenzo's parents refuse to accept the limitations of current treatments and begin to research possible alternatives on their own. They spend most of their time at home caring for their son or poring over research reports in the library. They can afford a home care nurse, but Michaela Odone, played by Susan Sarandon, angrily fires one nurse because she suggests that Lorenzo should be hospitalized or placed in hospice care. Any suggestion that the Odones should consider institutionalization or palliative care provokes Michaela's wrath. She throws her sister out of the house and even slaps her husband, Augusto Odone, played by Nick Nolte. While angrily confronting the professionals on the case, the Odones develop a treatment called "Lorenzo's Oil," which they believe reverses some of the neurological damage caused by ALD.

The imagery of the film explicitly invokes Christian iconography and martyrdom. Lorenzo is identified with the crucified Christ, suffering to save others; Michaela is the saint. In a cathedral scene the covering is removed from a statue of the Virgin Mary holding the Christ child. A later scene portrays Michaela holding Lorenzo in a similar pose. The film closes with images of angels and cameo shots of healthy boys who say that they have ALD but are doing well because of Lorenzo's Oil. Later developments have shown that Lorenzo's Oil is not effective in all cases (Jones 2000). Although the film is compelling and the Odones were remarkable parents and advocates, ordinary caregivers might see their own efforts as pitifully meager in comparison.

Marvin's Room (1996) offers another image of the saintly caregiver with a direct comparison between the "good" sister and the "bad" one. Bessie, played by Diane Keaton, has been caring for her father (Marvin) and aunt for two decades. Her sister, Lee, played by Meryl Streep, is the rebel in the family who refused to have anything to do with her father when he became ill several years earlier. The family is brought together, however, when Bessie is diagnosed with leukemia and reaches out to Lee and her nephews to ask if they would consider being donors for a bone marrow transplant. There is no match, and Bessie must face her death. Lee resists taking on the caregiver role. In one scene Bessie's doctor, played by Robert De Niro, automatically assumes that Lee will stay on to take care of Bessie as well as her father and aunt. Lee is offended and distraught at the implication, insisting that she cannot give up her life to take care of her sister, father, and aunt.

While Lee continues to resist the caregiver role, Bessie refuses any help with laundry or other tasks because she is so used to doing them. The climactic scene occurs when Bessie tells Lee that she has been so lucky in her life to have had the opportunity to spend so many years caring for her father and aunt. She has gained so much, she says, not just because they love her but because she loves them. Apparently, none of the other choices she might have made—career or marriage or both—would have brought her so much joy. Lee is so moved by this display of saintliness that she starts to take over the tasks of caregiving. This scene from the movie was presented to a conference on caregiving to show the rewards of caregiving and how lucky caregivers should feel to have this opportunity for spiritual growth. Yet one experienced caregiver found its message infuriating and wrote an essay to express her rage (Bendetson 1997).

The Eroticized Caregiver

Caregiving is not inherently romantic, although illness does not necessarily diminish or eliminate romantic feelings. There are films in which characters continue their romantic and sexual attachments despite illness or disability, such as the classic two-hanky movie *Love Story* (1970). The genre we emphasize in this section, however, are films in which the illness itself brings the partners together and creates the sexual bond. In *Love! Valour! Compassion!* (1997), a movie based on the play by Terrence McNally, eight gay men who make up a group of weekenders at a lovely country home are all involved romantically with one or another of their group. But it is the relationship between Buzz, played by Jason Alexander, and James, played by John Glover (in a twin role), which most clearly illustrates this theme.

In several scenes the growing attachment between Buzz, who is HIV-positive, and James, who has AIDS, is shown through Buzz's gentle bathing and touching of James's Kaposi's sarcoma lesions. Buzz's joy at finding love, only to face losing it through James's impending death, is sensitively portrayed. Buzz sees in James what he will become and is both angry and comforted. Would these two have found each other such compatible partners if the disease were not present? The film does not give us any clues about their attraction to each other beyond their shared experience with AIDS and as caregiver and care recipient.

Another film in which sex plays an even more essential role is *Coming Home,* a 1978 anti–Vietnam War movie. Jane Fonda plays Sally, a woman married to Bob, a Marine captain, played by Bruce Dern. While Bob is overseas, Sally volunteers at a local veterans' hospital and meets Luke, an angry paralyzed veteran, played by Jon Voight. She begins an affair with Luke (with explicit sex scenes), until Bob returns, emotionally traumatized by the war. Bob threatens Luke and Sally with a bayoneted rifle, and Luke leaves Sally to her husband. Bob, however, cannot live with his memories and swims out into the surf, presumably to his death. In this movie both Bob and Luke are grievously wounded, but it is Luke, wounded in body but a symbol of antiwar sentiment, who is the erotic figure. Again, would Sally and Luke have become involved if Luke had not been paralyzed? The film does not tell us.

A final movie in this genre is *Dying Young* (1991), in which Julia Roberts plays Hilary, a young woman whose life seems to have no purpose until she takes a job as a paid caregiver to Victor (played by Campbell Scott), also young but wealthy and educated. He is suffering from leukemia (the favorite film disease) and under the pressure of a domineering father. With no training at all, and after bumbling attempts to help Victor after his chemotherapy, Hilary finds creative ways to improve his health, nutrition, and outlook on life. When Victor's health improves, they drive to Mendocino for a change in scenery. At one point in Victor's most debilitated moments, Hilary had slept in his bed. Now Victor comes to her bed for sex. The scene can be interpreted as true love finding expression or as a not-so-subtle sexual ploy. In either case Victor's neediness and illness attract Hilary, giving her both a purpose in life and a rich partner, albeit one who will die young.

The More-or-Less Realistic Caregiver

Few films approach caregiving realistically, even considering the vast scope of caregiving situations in which people find themselves. Some films, however, do show some aspects of caregiving more or less realistically. Certainly, film is a medium in which the emotional aspects of caregiving—sadness, loss, grief, satisfaction, better or worsened relationships—can be and often are movingly portrayed. This emphasis on feelings can lead to the conclusion that caregiving is only an emotional experience, not a complex, hands-on, and managerial job.

In this genre *Iris* (2001) stands out. Based on the book *Elegy for Iris*, British literary critic John Bayley's memoir about his wife, the noted philosopher and novelist Iris Murdoch, and her descent into Alzheimer disease. With a stellar three Academy Award–nominated cast (Judi Dench and Jim Broadbent playing the elder Iris and John and Kate Winslet and Hugh Bonneville playing their younger selves), the movie does not flinch from showing Iris's confusion, childlike behavior, and growing dependence on her husband. From a caregiver's perspective Bayley is shown as totally (perhaps overly) devoted to a woman who had, by living an independent intellectual and sexual life during their marriage, never quite become his equal partner. Their prior lack of talent for domestic order takes on new meaning as Iris deteriorates. One can imagine a conscientious social worker, had one been on the scene, calling for protective services to clean up the mess. But, despite his growing frustration and despair, Bayley refused help until the very end—not exactly the best message to send to struggling caregivers. Still, in the portrayal of Iris's and John's losses—as well as the basic humanity and loving ties that remain—this is an unusual movie

One True Thing (1998), based on the novel by Anna Quindlen, is also more realistic than most movies. That is not surprising, since Quindlen's novel drew from her own experience caring for her dying mother. The plot revolves around the relationship between Ellen, an ambitious young journalist played by Renée Zellweger; her dying mother, Kate, played by Meryl Streep; and her self-centered father, George, played by William Hurt. George's pressure on Ellen to give up her job and take over her mother's care, while he continues with his academic career, is a variation on a theme that many caregivers experience. One brief but telling scene brings up the conflict between caregiving and the workplace. In an attempt to secure a substantial leave of absence to care for her mother, Ellen tells her editor at a trendy New York magazine about her mother's illness. Instead of offering sympathy, he responds, "Ellen, a sick mother gets you three weeks sick leave and a very nice flower arrangement and that's it."

Through Streep's convincing performance the debilitating ravages of illness are graphically portrayed. One particularly wrenching scene occurs when Kate can no longer get out of the bathtub and calls Ellen to help her. While this film has many moments that will ring true to caregivers, the family's spacious home and obvious affluence also allow a focus on the emotional trials that Ellen undergoes in learning to appreciate her mother more and to recognize her father's weaknesses.

In other films realism is a side story. For example, in *As Good as It Gets* (1997) the main plot concerns the relationship among Melvin, an irascible, obsessive-compulsive writer, played by Jack Nicholson; Carol, a waitress who tolerates his peculiarities; and Simon, a gay painter who is Melvin's neighbor. Carol, portrayed by Helen Hunt, is a single mother taking care of a young son with chronic asthma. As one of his steps toward more humane behavior, Melvin pays for a doctor to come to Carol's home to examine the boy, who has been denied treatment by Carol's HMO. In an exchange that generated audience applause, Carol says to the doctor, "Fucking HMO bastard pieces of shit!" After Carol apologizes for her outburst, the doctor replies: "That's okay. Actually, I think that's their technical name."

Conclusion

How should we view films that ostensibly portray family caregiving? Sometimes with tears, sometimes with laughter, and sometimes with anger. It is perhaps asking too much of a commercial medium to reflect reality, especially when there is no single reality that expresses the range of caregiver situations and emotions. And perhaps caregivers do not wish to see reality when they go to the movies; reality is all too present in their lives.

Still, caregivers should not be held to impossible standards, the saintly version, or perceived as abusers, the Gothic version. A Caregiver's Review of Current Movies, with ratings by numbers of pill bottles, might be a useful tool for caregivers and professionals alike, to point out what seems true to life and what is absurd or simply misinformed.

Caregivers also tend to see caregiving even when the movie is about something totally different. One of us (C.L.) took a break from caregiving to see a much-praised movie, *Crouching Tiger, Hidden Dragon,* precisely because it was an escapist movie, fantastic and foreign. Yet, in its portrayal of Chinese women warriors wielding swords in utterly impossible displays of martial arts, she saw herself: a caregiver always fighting "the system," always wielding whatever weapons she has at her command, always alert for the danger lurking in the shadows. What could be further from the filmmaker's intent? Yet in some ways this describes caregiving more honestly than the films that approach the theme directly.

REFERENCES

Bendetson, J. (1997, Apr. 13). "I Am More than Hands." *New York Times Magazine,* 96.
Dans, Peter. (2000). *Doctors in the Movies: Boil the Water and Just Say Aah.* Bloomington, Ill.: Medi-Ed Press.
Denzin, Norman. (1995). *The Cinematic Society: The Voyeur's Gaze.* Thousand Oaks, Calif.: Sage.
———. (1991). *Hollywood Shot by Shot: Alcoholism in American Cinema.* New York: Aldine de Gruyter.
Jones, A. H. (2000, Oct.). "Medicine and the Movies: *Lorenzo's Oil* at Century's End." *Annals of Internal Medicine* 133(7):67–71.

Part IV / Bridging the Gap among Cultures

on how the burdens of care which family members are expected to assume raise troubling questions about the justice of our health care system (Smith 1993; Nelson and Nelson 1995; Levine and Zuckerman 2000). What emerges from these discussions, among other things, is a picture of the family as system of care whose values, attitudes, and behaviors distinguish it conceptually, ethically, and emotionally from other sorts of caring relationships.

Health professionals' increasing dependence on family members for patient care and management is sustainable only if their mutual dependence is accompanied by mutual respect. Mutual respect, in turn, depends upon the recognition that the institutions of family and medicine embody distinctive conceptions of care and sets of values, each valid within its own domain (Nelson and Nelson 1995). Here the contributions of family ethics and medical ethics are both important, for each articulates and defends the values peculiar to its system of care. The critical question for health professionals, families, and society is whether and to what extent these values can be integrated in a coherent ethic of care.

This chapter takes up this question. I hope to show that such an integration is at least a theoretical possibility and to suggest some respects in which it can be achieved. The sort of integration that I believe is desirable involves a *partnership* between those who provide care, not a blurring of their respective functions. The distinction between the role of medical professional and the role of family member can be blurred in different ways. One occurs when medical staff attempt to fill the void created by the absence of a supportive and intimate family, another when the physician attempts to provide ongoing care for his or her family members. In both instances there is a failure to respect the differences between medical care and family care, and, however well intentioned this merging of roles might be, ultimately neither the patient nor the health professional is well served.

The kind of collaboration I envision between medicine and the family recognizes and respects the distinctive character, strengths, and limitations of each form of caregiving. But, for this collaboration to become a reality, misconceptions about the family must first be dispelled.

Misconceptions about the Family

The effort to articulate a coherent ethic of care faces significant obstacles, including misconceptions about the moral nature of the family. These mis-

CHAPTER NINE

Integrating Medicine and the Family

Toward a Coherent Ethic of Care

Jeffrey Blustein

The family is a critical medical resource for health professionals. Family members are called upon to make or be involved in treatment decisions for their incapacitated relatives because consent is needed for diagnostic tests or procedures, because professionals feel they do not know the patient well enough to make decisions without family input, and for various other reasons. Health professionals also turn to family members to provide long-term care once patients are discharged from the acute care setting. In these ways medical practice acknowledges and utilizes the reality that patients, embedded within a network of family relationships, do not as a rule interact with the health care system as isolated individuals.

Only within the past decade or so, however, has thinking about the family among medical ethicists begun to catch up with a medical practice that relies so heavily on family involvement. Ethicists have turned the spotlight on the role that families should and do play in medical decision making for capacitated as well as incapacitated adults and on the morally significant impact that treatment decisions have on the lives and interests of family members and have even called into question medicine's traditional patient-centered ethic (Hardwig 1990; Blustein 1993; Kuczewski 1996). They have also reflected on what makes the family a distinctively valuable form of human association and conceptions include the idea that the family is always a unified entity, that concern for oneself always equals morally unjustified selfishness, and that the obligations family members have to care for one another are firmly rooted in biology.

The family is a unit

Most discussions about the family start with the assertion that the family is a unit, and in some sense that is true. Some families, however, are merely aggregates of individuals for whom family membership carries little or no moral or emotional significance. They are "family" only from a biological or legalistic standpoint; what is missing is emotional identification with the good of the family as such and a valuing of the family not only for what it does but also for what it is. The interests pursued by such family members are self-regarding: they have their own private goals, which are either competing or independent but not complementary. By contrast, in intimate, loving families the family has interests and goals that are not reducible to those of its individual members. In these families individual members share some common goals and accommodate differing goals held by others. They derive meaning from their membership because family relationships are intrinsically valuable to them. These features distinguish families that are genuine communities from families that are made up of aggregated individuals.

Although the mostly highly prized and often envied families are genuine communities, we should not exaggerate the extent of harmony even there. It is not necessary for community that there be complete identity of all ends and unanimity on all matters among its members but only that whatever conflicts and disagreements may arise are managed cooperatively. Absolute harmony is rare and not the norm even in tightly knit, well-functioning families. Allen Buchanan and Dan Brock are emphatic in their rejection of this kind of communitarian thinking: "To speak of the family as having its own goals and purposes and to speak of the familial perspective and familial objectives is to engage in dangerous reification" (1989, 236). Their criticism may go too far in the opposite direction, but, interpreted as a warning, the point is well taken. Reference to the family's interest or familial objectives is all too likely to mask the way in which more powerful members impose their will on more vulnerable ones. Even in loving families, in which compromises may be made for the good of the family and disagreements may be muted, individuals have distinct and possibly conflicting interests and goals.

Most leading theorists of justice have neglected this fact. As Susan Moller Okin notes, it is typical of contemporary theories of justice to treat the family as a "nonpolitical" entity and thereby tacitly to rule out the application of principles of justice to it. In one way or another, she claims, almost all current theories "take mature, independent human beings as the subjects of their theories without any mention of how they got to be that way" (1989, 9). Thus, these theorists assume that family exists but do not examine the distribution of rights and responsibilities, benefits and burdens, within it in light of whatever standards of justice they propose.

Their neglect of the family does not mean that theorists of justice believe the family is a completely harmonious community, without internal dissension or disagreement. But it amounts to much the same thing, since, by failing to extend their principles to the household, they mask the separateness of family members and their distinctive interests. Medical practice too often reflects a similar indifference in making decisions about and arranging for the care of patients and so tacitly treats the family as if it were a single undifferentiated entity. This is "dangerous reification" indeed. To the extent that this happens, the bonds of family cohesion may actually be weakened and the welfare of patients who rely on their families for care jeopardized.

Self-concern is selfishness

The second myth is that families must sacrifice all for one another, and that failing to do so is unconscionable selfishness. In a well-known criticism of impartialist moral theory Bernard Williams (1973) argues that both utilitarianism and Kantianism impose unreasonable demands on individuals. These theories, he claims, insist that agents make decisions from an impartial point of view, in abstraction from their personal circumstances, and that they be prepared to sacrifice even those projects with which they most closely identify and which give them a reason for living. The demand that they do so, Williams contends, constitutes an attack on their integrity.

Whether or not one accepts Williams's critique of moral theory, my point is that widespread expectations concerning the extent to which family members should sacrifice for one another and, in particular, for sick members who require ongoing care are often unreasonable in just this way. Societal norms dictate that, as a mark of genuine affection and concern, family members (and especially female members) set aside whatever competing projects and commitments they may have and devote themselves entirely to the care of their needy loved ones. Anything less than complete dedication to their welfare, it is assumed, is not a way for caregivers to preserve their integrity but reflects self-indulgence at the expense of those who need care and an objectionable expression of selfishness. Caregivers who are singled out for praise and awards, even by caregiving organizations, are invariably those who have given up everything they previously valued (and even the best interests of others in their family) to provide care. (For an example, see *Caregivers USA News* 2002.) Because these expectations of self-sacrifice are internalized by those who bear the burdens of care and measured against public approbation for total sacrifice, even the temptation to pursue independent interests is likely to be accompanied by tremendous guilt.

Selfless devotion to the needs of a sick family member may be morally admirable, but saintliness of this sort should not be the norm by which we assess the contribution of caregivers. The problem of integrity here is analogous to the one Williams discusses in a different context: as a society, we do not give caregivers, especially women, permission to limit for self-regarding reasons the care they give to sick or needy loved ones. The costs of this disregard of caregiver integrity will become more apparent as the responsibilities and burdens of health care continue to be shifted to families.

Obligations of care are rooted in biology

Except for marriage, the facts about familial relationships that ground special obligations to family members are often thought to involve biological connection centrally. This is the third myth about families. Families, it is said, are nonconsensual. We do not choose our family circumstances, and the obligations that arise from family membership do not resemble the obligations that arise from contracts or promises. This is often explained in the following way: our obligations to family members are based on something distinctive about familial relationships as such, and what is distinctive about them is their grounding in biology. We do not choose our biology, but it morally constrains us nonetheless. This is a commonsense view, but it quickly collapses under the weight of its unattractive implications. No doubt biology has some role to play in the story about the grounds of special obligations to family members. Yet the inescapability of the facts of biology does not render such facts morally dispositive or even morally important. Imposing obligations of care on family members merely because they are biologically related to the patient, without taking into account other aspects or dimensions of their relationship, is not only morally dubious but also likely to breed hostility and resentment in those who feel burdened by an unwelcome responsibility.

Whatever the grounds of special familial obligations may be, it is vital to protect and foster conditions of intimacy in which family members are motivated to fulfill their obligations and do not perceive them as excessively burdensome and unfair. As Carol Levine (1998) reminds us, family members more often than not want to do their best for one of their own who is ill, but even the best of intentions can be eroded by practices that are insensitive to the psychological and other costs of caregiving. In particular, appeal to biology can too easily become an excuse for "dumping" caregiving responsibilities on family members, an impediment to the sort of collaboration between medicine and family which gives due recognition to the interests of patients and family members alike.

Clarifying the Values of Medicine

Since I am interested in exploring whether a coherent ethic of care incorporating the values of medicine and family is possible, I turn next to consider medicine's values and the extent to which they can or cannot accommodate the values of family. The values that we associate with medicine and family are not solely moral in nature. Medicine is grounded in the biological sciences and is characterized in part by adherence to the norms of scientific inquiry; families have enormous historical, psychological, and emotional value for their members. Important though they are for an adequate understanding of medicine and family, these are nonmoral values and as such are not the focus of my investigation. The line between moral and nonmoral is not always easy to draw, of course. Values may have moral as well as nonmoral dimensions, and even among moral philosophers there is some controversy over what makes something a specifically "moral" value. I shall assume, however, that the distinction between moral and nonmoral is sufficiently clear to convey what I mean by the values of medicine and family.

One way to articulate the moral values of medicine is in terms of the moral principles widely accepted by health professionals as guidelines for medical practice: autonomy, beneficence, and justice. The principle of autonomy requires respect for the capacity of self-determining agents to determine their own destiny; they are to be accorded the right to choose their own vision of the good and act accordingly, as long as this does not violate the rights of others. The principle of beneficence enjoins health care professionals to do no harm to others, to protect them from harm, and to promote their welfare. Justice, the third principle, requires fairness in distributing benefits and burdens and resolving disputes through fair procedures.

Thus stated, these principles do not necessarily conflict with what is distinctively valuable about family relationships. Properly understood, respect for autonomy, for example, does not mean that the patient is viewed as an isolated atom, without any ties of affection and obligation to intimate others. Nor does the principle of beneficence entail a narrow view of patient welfare, in which the welfare of family members has no place. Like all abstract principles, the basic principles of medical ethics require interpretation if they are to guide action usefully, and they can be interpreted in ways that recognize the importance that family has, or should have, for its members.

Nevertheless, some might still perceive a threat to family relationships from the guiding norms of medicine. A concern might be that the principles of medical ethics do not give sufficient moral weight to "the personalities and life situations of specific family members" (Nelson and Nelson 1995, 68), since the clinical worldview of health professionals is such that they tend "to treat all clients in a like manner, regardless of each client's unique personal situation" (Darling 1991, 140). Yet it would be rash to suppose that, since the clinical perspective of the health professional tends to be impersonal in this way, the principles of medical ethics cannot adequately accommodate particularity. The ethical principles governing the practice of medicine are open to interpretations that are not reflected in the dominant norms of the culture of medicine.

Concern about the alleged individualism of medicine, alluded to earlier, deserves further comment. *Individualism,* of course, is a notoriously ambiguous term. Interpreted in one way, individualism is the ideology of self-reliance and mutual independence, which, from a sociological point of view, has its roots in our peculiarly American frontier experience. In its Kantian version, however, individualism is the view that the autonomous agent is an end in himself, of incomparable worth and not to be treated merely as a means to the ends of others. Insofar as the individualism of medicine is understood in this way, there is no conflict between medicine's values and family values, since being a member of a family does not nullify this basic moral entitlement.

The conflict arises when individualism is interpreted as implying that self-sufficiency, independence, and separation from others are goals worth pursuing, perhaps preeminently so. Insofar as these values shape medical practice, the patient is detached from relationship with others, and family relationships are taken into account merely as aspects of the self-interested feelings of individuals. Lucy Candib describes the problem: "declaring patients to be autonomous [interpreted as implying these values] recasts them as fictitiously independent actors rather than as the emotional and social beings we all are" (1995, 128).

This is not how medicine has to be. There is nothing intrinsic to the nature or goals of medicine which requires this particular interpretation of medical values. But an almost obsessive patient-centered orientation in contemporary medicine is undeniable. Part of the explanation is related to the widespread rejection of *medical paternalism* as the governing principle in relations between health professionals and their patients. Paternalism gives the physician complete discretion in terms of how much and what is disclosed to patients and what medical interventions are pursued. Recognition of a patient's rights to active participation in the decision-making process is a necessary and important corrective to this power imbalance. In recent years the focus on patients' rights has intensified as patients have come to be regarded as *consumers* of medical services. This notion, borrowed from the marketplace, brings a set of normative assumptions which distorts our conception of the proper practice of medicine and fuels ever-increasing demands by patients for various medical services. Arguably, the pendulum has swung from one extreme to the other, from the regime of medical paternalism to the era of consumer sovereignty.

The consumerist mentality that drives so much of health care today is not confined to the medical domain, of course. Consumerism is one of the hallmarks of contemporary American life, frequently cited by social critics as a symptom of the moral degeneration of our culture. But its effects are not always pernicious: they depend on the kind of goods consumed and on whether consumerism is confined to those spheres of social life in which it is appropriate to distribute goods on this basis. For various reasons, not the least of which is its potential damaging effects on the family, medicine's adoption of the values of consumerism is profoundly disturbing.

Thomas Murray eloquently describes the deep differences between market values and the values of family life:

Liberty and the model of the autonomous, self-interested individual so dear to
economic theory are a flimsy foundation on which to build an ethic of the family...The values we think of as crucial to family life tend either to be found only
in the context of relationships—love, loyalty, affection, trust, care—or, given our
social natures, to depend utterly on a foundation of good, enduring relationships—identity, self-confidence, maturation...In the market, relationships are
secondary to the fair and efficient exchange of goods and services: I deal with you
not because I prize the intrinsic value of our relationship but because you have
something I want, and vice versa. (1996, 19, 24)

Patients come to physicians and other health professionals for medical assistance, for the cure and prevention of illness and disease, or, when a cure is not
possible, for help in living with residual pain, discomfort, or disability. The
physician-patient relationship, once established, is multifaceted and remarkable for its peculiar combination of intimacy and professionalism. To the extent that medicine embraces the values of the marketplace and treats patients
as consumers, the complex relationship between patient and physician is im-
poverished:

One impact of consumerism on medicine has been the loss of relationship; in the
proliferation of medical marketplace jargon, doctoring is now a product to be
packaged, marketed, and provided. Contracts between doctor and patient situate
the transaction in commercial terms. (Candib 1995, 132)

The point for our purposes is this: medicine contributes to the erosion of
the values of family and the moral relationships between the patient and
other family members when medicine embraces marketplace values that then
determine how it interacts with families.

Should medicine care about these things? Medicine is a moral enterprise
and, as such, must be sensitive to the broader ethical and social implications
of its practice. This is recognized by those who argue that, from the standpoint of social justice, the ethic of exclusive fidelity to the interests of one's
patients is morally irresponsible. It requires no radical conceptual departure
from the norms of medicine to bring family values within the ambit of its
concerns.

The threat to these values, I suspect, comes less from the values of medicine than from the values of the marketplace, which have deformed both the
family and the practice of medicine. If so, then there is reason to hope that

medicine can work collaboratively with families to ensure adequate care for patients and the continued viability of the families to which they belong. Even with a different conceptualization of the values of medicine, the culture of medicine and the culture of families will remain distinct: medicine cannot care for patients the way families can, and vice versa. But there are possibilities for a refashioning of medical values and a change of medical culture which diminish the antagonism between these two social institutions.

Eric Cassell's writings on the culture of medicine suggest one way this might be done: by making the philosophy and practice of primary care medicine "the foundation for twenty-first- century doctoring" (1997, 3). According to Cassell, this philosophy involves a richer understanding of what it means to be focused on the patient: "the physician [is] focused not on this patient to the exclusion of everything else, but on *this* patient as a person who must always exist in relation to others and to a community" (120). The focus on the patient-in-relation brings the family out of the ethical shadows, so to speak, and permits a more serious consideration of its peculiar values and the mutual responsibilities of family members. If the patient exists in relation to family, then the family exists in relation to the patient, and its character and the burdens of care it shoulders must be taken seriously.

Mixing the Functions of Medicine and Family

We can further clarify and contrast the values and defining features of family and medicine by considering two problematic situations in which the distinction between medicine and family is not maintained. In one, medical professionals attempt to take the place of family; in the other, family members attempt to function as medical professionals.

Medical staff as family

With very few exceptions the day of the all-knowing, ever-present family doctor has long passed. In this era of managed care and frequent changes in employer-sponsored health insurance plans, it is becoming increasingly rare even for patients who can afford private insurance to establish close, ongoing relationships with particular health care providers. The millions in our society who do not have adequate insurance or who are uninsured often receive care, if they receive care at all, in chaotic emergency rooms, which are set up to process as many people as possible as rapidly as possible. But in some circumstances relationships can develop between patients and health providers which involve a level of personal involvement which may lead providers to think of themselves as family. This is particularly likely when such relationships are established with patients who either have no family at all or come from dysfunctional families.

One such circumstance is described in a survey of the attitudes of emergency nurses toward "heavy users" of emergency department (ED) services (Malone 1996). Because these patients are seen often enough and long enough for nurses to gain some familiarity with more than their immediate medical problems, staff frequently reports becoming attached to these patients as if they were somehow "like family." For the patient being known in this way is often at least as important as getting medical attention. The fact that ED staff members remember even a few small details of the patient's life means that he is "not just 'any patient': he stands out as worth remembering something about, and he is therefore able to show up as a member of the ED family" (181).

It is understandable that in some situations health professionals develop a special attachment to particular patients and form a strong bond with them. It is also understandable that health care providers should think of themselves as family in some cases: relationships between patients and health professionals are so tenuous and fleeting these days that it is not surprising if health providers and patients alike sometimes interpret expressions of more than purely professional concern in this way. But in their role as health providers they can never actually *be* family, and it is dangerous for them as well as for patients to suppose otherwise. Patients may come to expect a level and continuity of care which the staff cannot possibly provide, and staff may feel overburdened and resentful of patients because they demand so much.

One difference between medical staff and family has to do with the degree of intimacy. The relationship between nurse and patient or physician and patient is essentially a professional one, and a professional relationship is an example of a *role relation* (Blustein 1991, 157–60). Role relationships need not be cold, unfriendly, and uncaring; indeed, these are characteristics for which we rightly criticize health professionals. Moreover, there are some caregivers with respect to whom the line between the personal and the professional is not as sharply drawn as this: boundary issues frequently arise in the case of home health aides, for example. But patients and medical staff relate to each other as occupiers of roles and so engage in more or less narrowly prescribed reciprocal behaviors.

Because their interactions are circumscribed and limited, the extent of their familiarity with each other is necessarily limited as well. Intimate knowledge of the patient's life, character, and desires is lacking; knowledge is sought primarily for its usefulness in fulfilling the role. In a family, or at least a well-functioning family, by contrast, interactions are holistic and multifaceted. On the basis of shared common interests and/or a long shared history, family members develop bonds of intimacy, and this intimacy alters relationships in at least two ways. First, intimates know each other in a deeply personal and highly particularized way, and this knowledge offers them special possibilities of mutual support and concern. Second, their lives and interests become closely intertwined, so that the happiness of one is bound up with and contingent on the happiness of the other. The distinction I am drawing here can be put succinctly as follows: we prize families chiefly (but not exclusively) for the special goods of intimacy they convey, whereas we prize professional relationships chiefly (but again not exclusively) for the particular services they provide.

Another important and closely related difference between health professionals and family members concerns the nature and ground of their respective obligations. The obligations of medical providers are relatively determinate prescriptions; those of family members are more open-ended in that family members are called upon to be responsive to changes in one another's needs, desires, and circumstances. Further, although the relationship between health professional and patient is not merely contractual (Candib 1995, 129 ff), it is nevertheless true that the obligations of medical providers are more akin to those that arise from contracts and promises than are the obligations of family members. There are fairly definite conditions for entering into a valid contract and legitimately terminating it, and obligations that arise out of contract cease when the contract is no longer binding. In the case of the family, however, it is considerably more difficult to specify the conditions under which family members no longer have obligations to one another. Much more so than providers and patients, "family members are stuck with each other," as the Nelsons aptly put it (1995, 75). Moral relationships among family members can certainly be strained by indifference, betrayal, and violence, but the threshold that must be passed before they are dissolved is typically extremely high.

Family member as family physician

Many medical societies discourage physicians from treating their own family members. For example, the policy of the American College of Physicians reflects the widespread belief that this practice compromises the physician's ability to deliver good medical care: "Physicians should avoid treating themselves, close friends, or members of their own families...If a physician does treat a close friend, family member, or employee out of necessity, the patient should be transferred to another physician as soon as it is practical. Otherwise, requests for care on the part of employees, family members, or friends should be resolved by assisting them in obtaining appropriate care. Fulfilling the role of informed and loving adviser, however, is not precluded" (1998, 582). The American Medical Association takes a similar position regarding immediate family members, as does the Canadian Medical Association.

Although having "a doctor in the house" may seem to offer many advantages to patients, in general it is unwise for physicians to undertake the care of family members and other intimates (La Puma 1991; La Puma and Priest 1992; Tulsky et al. 1999). Even serving as surrogate decision maker evokes clinical and ethical tensions (Issa 2002). One reason has to do with the greater rigidity that moral rules have in their application to patients as compared with family members. Physicians have little latitude to act in disregard of the moral requirements that pertain to the physician-patient relationship. They are supposed to inform capable patients fully about the risks and benefits of treatment, to tell patients the truth unless there is compelling reason to believe that immediate and grave harm will result, and to respect patient confidentiality. Compliance with these requirements is often the only ground of trust which patients have in their physicians, and that trust may be badly damaged if patients find out that important information has been withheld from them, that they have not been told the truth, or that confidentiality has been breached. Understandably, patients are not as a rule terribly understanding and accepting of these acts of noncompliance with physician obligations.

By contrast, family members normally do not expect from one another such strict compliance with moral requirements, and they tend to be more forgiving of one another's moral lapses. This is so because in families there is a basis for trust which does not exist in the physician-patient relationship, namely, mutual love and affection. Family members have greater reserves of good feeling to draw on than patients do and so give one another greater latitude to interpret moral requirements and even to act in disregard of them (Deigh 1989).

A physician who undertakes the care of family members is therefore in a deeply conflictual moral position. As a physician, he is required and expected to adhere strictly to certain moral rules in dealings with patients. But, as a family member, these requirements are greatly relaxed. If, for example, he withholds the truth regarding a diagnosis from a family member, he may be acting appropriately as a family member but inappropriately as a physician. Which relationship is the primary one for purposes of deciding what action is or is not morally permissible or obligatory?

A second difficulty with occupying dual relationships has to do with how open a family member is willing to be with another family member who doubles as her physician. In this connection there is another romantic myth about the close, loving family which needs to be dispelled, namely, that its members have no inhibitions about sharing everything about themselves. This, it may be claimed, is one thing that distinguishes ideal families from dysfunctional families, mere acquaintanceships, and the highly impersonal relationships of everyday social life. But the contrast is too sharply drawn. Even within very loving and healthy families there are limits to intimacy: personal boundaries are established, some private information may be too sensitive or embarrassing to probe, certain secrets might not be shared even with those we love. Complete baring of body and soul is neither a requirement of genuine intimacy nor an ideal of family life to which we should aspire.

Personal medical or health-related information that individuals might be uncomfortable divulging to family members, or parts of their bodies they might be uncomfortable exposing to them, they may be comfortable revealing to a physician, precisely because he or she is a physician and not a member of the family. The relationships are different in part because of differences in the norms and expectations regarding appropriate patient self-disclosure to family members and physicians. (There are also differences in norms and expectations regarding appropriate physician self-disclosure to patients and members of his or her family.) If physicians respect their family members' feelings in such matters, as they will want to do, they might not be able to get a complete medical history or do a thorough physical examination, and this will compromise their ability to provide good medical care.

In the setting of home care there is an analogous problem. Family members who are not trained as medical professionals function as *informal* caregivers for their ill relatives. In this role they must cross personal boundaries that, as family members, they would ordinarily not trespass out of respect for the other's privacy and sense of personal dignity. They must come in contact with and manage the most intimate and private details of the patient's bodily functioning on a daily basis. The argument against physicians treating family members—namely, that there are limits to what even family members should have to disclose to and demand of one another—should lead us to take seriously, indeed more seriously than we do, the caregiving burdens we place on family members. The ethical concern here can be partly couched in terms of fairness or justice, that is, how caregiving responsibilities are apportioned among family members and others. But the concern more particularly has to do with a potential consequence of such allocation which is internal to the family, such as the erosion of personal boundaries in the face of ongoing needs for care.

These observations about physicians treating family members point to the following general problem: providing good and appropriate care depends on the physician's ability to be objective, and, when physicians treat their own family members, emotional involvement interferes with objectivity. Physicians make objective decisions based on physical findings, laboratory data, and symptoms; emotional detachment is necessary in order to consider patients and their problems objectively. If physicians are too close to their patients, as they are likely to be if the patients are family members, their professional judgment may be impaired. This loss of objectivity can manifest itself in overtesting and overtreatment as well as undertesting and undertreatment of family members as compared with unrelated patients (La Puma 1992, 1811).

One must be careful here, however, not to posit a false dichotomy between objectivity and subjectivity, to suppose that emotional involvement (i.e., "subjectivity") is necessarily antithetical to fair, careful, and temperate appraisal of another's actions, needs, and interests ("objectivity"). Indeed, depending on the situation, emotional detachment may prevent one from being able to make such judgments about another person. Max Deutscher argues against the conventional notions of objectivity and subjectivity: "One must name the emotional involvement before considering a proposition such as that objectivity is impaired by emotional involvement...It is because we are delighted, distressed, shocked, absorbed by and in the doings and matters which happen to someone we love that conventional myth has it that those who love lose their objectivity. This is simply part of the conventional, false cliché that to be objective is to be uncommitted, impersonal, uninvolved, moderate, impartial, calm and unemotional" (1983, 60–61).

As applied to physicians treating their families, the point is a simple one but easily forgotten: physicians should generally avoid treating their family members because doing so interferes with the kind of objectivity which is required of physicians, not because universally, or even typically, affection and close ties make fair and accurate judgment impossible. In some important respects family members who have a long history of intimate association with the patient may know him or her better than the physician, whose dealings with the patient are largely professional in nature.

In sum, the relationship between medical professional and patient, on the one hand, and family member and patient, on the other, differ in a number of significant ways. There are differences in the level and degree of intimacy possible, the durability and strictness of physician and family obligations, assumptions about appropriate patient self-disclosure, and the kinds of objective knowledge of the patient available to physician and family. An ethic of care which integrates the values of medicine and family should be one that recognizes and preserves these differences.

Bringing Family and Medicine Closer Together

In order to effect a genuine partnership between medicine and family, it is necessary to change current professional values and attitudes so that health professionals, particularly physicians, become more sensitive to and considerate of the needs of families, the burdens of family caregiving, and the distinctive ways in which families manage the care of their sick and disabled members. Beyond this, what specific forms of collaboration, what efforts at accommodation, are possible and desirable? One fairly radical suggestion, put forward by John Hardwig, is that in the area of medical decision making for capacitated adults it may be appropriate to empower the family to "make the treatment decision, with all competent family members whose lives will be affected participating" (1990, 9). I have critically discussed this proposal elsewhere (Blustein 1993). Another suggestion, which seems more promising, is to borrow elements of the philosophy and practice of palliative and hospice care and apply them more broadly to the care of patients who are not necessarily in the terminal phase of illness but who may be afflicted with a chronic illness or living with a permanently disabling condition.

In the United States hospice was imported from the British model as an alternative to the increasing medicalization and institutionalization of death. In an era when most patients died in institutions, surrounded by strangers who administered invasive and often futile life-prolonging interventions, hospice focused on providing comprehensive palliative care to terminally ill patients which addresses the physical, spiritual, and psychosocial dimensions of the dying process. In hospice care, however, emphasis is not only placed on providing the best quality of life for patients until death.

As John Finn and Ronald Schonwetter point out, "in hospice and palliative care, the patient and family comprise the unit of care. The patient is viewed not as a disease, but as a person who is a member of an entire family system. Hospice programs emphasize empowerment of patients and families...Hospice team members recognize the family's need for information, for help with practical matters, for assistance with decision making, and for ongoing discussions of their concerns" (1997, 10). The goal of hospice care is to alleviate the suffering of family members as well as terminally ill patients by providing support and guidance throughout the patient's illness and during the bereavement period.

Physicians practicing in palliative and hospice care settings collaborate with all members of an interdisciplinary team—nurses, home health aides, social workers, clergy, volunteers, and other specialized health care professionals—to ensure a comprehensive and coordinated response to the suffering of patients and their family members. Unlike acute care settings, where the patient's medical needs tend to be the exclusive focus of concern, hospice care attends to the impact of illness on all aspects of the patient's life, including the patient's family.

These features of hospice care make it a particularly helpful model for thinking about ways of integrating medicine and family and preserving valuable features of each. There is also strategic value in using it as a model: hospice is increasingly being recognized as an integral part of mainstream medicine. The success of palliative and hospice care depends on a number of factors that have more general application beyond end-of-life care. These include: involvement of family members in decision making; understanding of family dynamics by health providers; education of patients and their families about the disease process, available resources and how to access them, and what to expect in terms of the family's participation in care; ongoing primary care by attending physicians after hospital discharge; respectful consideration of the feelings and interests of family members; and effective communication with patients and families. To be sure, we should not minimize the significant regulatory, institutional, and other barriers to incorporating these elements of hospice care in medical practice generally. But, by advocating for their wider acceptance and working to overcome barriers to hospice care, we take an important practical step toward transforming an uneasy relationship into a partnership that harmonizes the values of medicine and family (American Medical Association, Council on Scientific Affairs 1993; Levine and Zuckerman 1999).

Physicians and other health professionals can advocate for patients and their families in other ways as well. They can educate family caregivers about how to interact with other professionals, what questions to ask, and when decisions should be challenged; they can give caregivers information about and work with them to secure needed services. In these and other ways health professionals become allies of the family in negotiating an often bewildering and unaccommodating health care system.

Conclusion

I have argued that the rise of consumerist values in medicine, and the attendant neglect of family and personal relationship, is not an inevitable outcome of a commitment to principles of autonomy and beneficence. Moreover, the language of the marketplace debases the deeply ethical traditions of medicine and is woefully inadequate to express its moral character. I have also argued that there are several misconceptions about the family which need to be dispelled if we are to arrive at an ethically defensible conception of *family values*. Further, the notion of family values as I have used the term presupposes no particular institutional form of the family and no marital or biological relationship between its members. What I have emphasized in my discussion of the family are the moral values of intimacy, long-term commitment, and personal caring. These values are expressed in family caregiving; the values of medicine are different from but not necessarily antithetical to them.

REFERENCES

American College of Physicians. (1998, Apr. 1). *Ethics Manual,* 4th ed. *Annals of Internal Medicine* 128(7):576–94.

American Medical Association, Council on Scientific Affairs. (1993). "Physicians and Family Caregivers: A Model for Partnership." *Journal of the American Medical Association* 269(10):1282–84.

Blustein, Jeffrey. (1991). *Care and Commitment: Taking the Personal Point of View.* New York: Oxford University Press.

———. (1993). "The Family in Medical Decision-Making." *Hastings Center Report* 23(3):6–13.

Buchanan, A. E. , and D. W. Brock. (1989). *Deciding for Others: The Ethics of Surrogate Decision Making.* New York: Cambridge University Press.

Candib, Lucy. (1995). *Medicine and the Family.* New York: Basic Books.

Caregivers USA News. (2002). "St. Louis Caregiver Honored." Accessed at http://www.atsh.org/news, Dec. 30.

Cassell, Eric J. (1997). *Doctoring: The Nature of Primary Care Medicine.* New York: Oxford University Press.

Darling, Rosalyn. (1991). "Parent-Professional Interaction: The Roots of Misunderstanding." In *The Family with a Handicapped Child,* ed. Milton Seligman, 2d ed. Boston: Allyn and Bacon.

Deigh, John. (1989). "Morality and Personal Relations." In *Person to Person,* ed. George Grahama and Hugh LaFollette. Philadelphia: Temple University Press.

Deutscher, Max. (1983). *Subjecting and Objecting.* Oxford: Blackwell.

Finn, John, and Ronald Schonwetter. (1997). "Hospice and Palliative Medicine: Philosophy, History, and Standards of Care." In American Academy of Hospice and Palliative Medicine (AAHPM), *Hospice and Palliative Medicine: Core Curriculum and Review Syllabus.*

Hardwig, John. (1990). "What about the Family?" *Hastings Center Report* 20(2): 9.

Issa, Amalia M. (2002). "Taking Off the White Coat: Can Family Members Who Are Physicians Be Good Surrogate Decision-Makers?" *Journal of the American Geriatric Society* 50:946–48.

La Puma, John, and Rush Priest. (1992, Apr. 1). "Is There a Doctor in the House?" *JAMA* 267(13): 1810–12.

La Puma, John, et al. (1991, Oct. 31). "When Physicians Treat Members of Their Own Families." *New England Journal of Medicine* 325(18):1290–94.

Levine, Carol. (1998). *Rough Crossings: Family Caregivers' Odyssey through the Health Care System.* New York: United Hospital Fund.

Levine, C., and C. Zuckerman. (1999). "The Trouble with Families: Toward an Ethic of Accommodation." *Annals of Internal Medicine* 130:148–52.

————. (2000). "Hands On, Hands Off: Why Health Care Professionals Depend on Families but Keep Them at Arm's Length." *Journal of Law, Medicine, and Ethics* 28(1):5–18.

Malone, Ruth. (1996, June). "Almost 'like Family': Emergency Nurses and 'Frequent Flyers."' *Journal of Emergency Nursing* 22(3):176–83.

Murray, Thomas H. (1996). *The Worth of a Child.* Berkeley: University of California Press.

Nelson, Hilde Lindemann, and James Lindemann Nelson. (1995). *The Patient in the Family.* New York: Routledge.

Okin, Susan Miller. (1989). *Justice, Gender, and the Family.* New York: Basic Books.

Tulsky, J. A., et al. (1999, Jan.). "Should Doctors Treat Their Relatives?" *ACP-ASIM Observer* 19(1):1–7.

Williams, Bernard. (1973). "A Critique of Utilitarianism." In *Utilitarianism For and Against,* ed. J. J. C. Smart and Bernard Williams. Cambridge: Cambridge University Press.

CHAPTER TEN

Project DOCC
A Parent-Directed Model for Educating
Pediatric Residents

Maggie Hoffman and Donna Jean Appell

We were three mothers with one thing in common: we were parents of children with special health care needs. Time and trials brought us closer as we were challenged by the needs of our families. We felt isolated from our communities and frustrated by the health care systems. We came together in June 1994 to create a new model for educating the pediatricians who take care of our children. These are our stories.

The Importance of Having a Pivotal Physician

In 1986 Donna Jean Appell gave birth to Ashley, who was diagnosed with albinism. When Ashley started trying to walk at the age of one, she became terribly bruised from her clumsy attempts. Donna felt that there was something more wrong than just albinism. And after a major struggle Ashley was eventually diagnosed with Hermansky-Pudlak syndrome (HPS). HPS is a very rare, autosomally recessive disease involving albinism, legal blindness, a platelet defect with a bleeding disorder, and a lysosomal ceroid accumulation disease. In an unusual progression of the disease Ashley became affected with the granulomatous inflammatory bowel disease associated with HPS before she was three years old.

On October 12, 1989, at 3:00 A.M. (but who recalls details!), Donna found Ashley's crib full of blood overflowing from her diaper. She left her four-month-old son with her husband and drove to the hospital. When they arrived, Ashley, limp from blood loss, was admitted to an intensive care unit. Hardly recognizable when the staff completed her workup, Ashley seemed to be hooked up to every piece of equipment they had. She was getting blood and bleeding all at the same time. Donna never forgot the doctors who admitted that they had no experience with HPS but who cared very much and would be willing to learn with her. Their honesty was the most comforting thing they could have ever shared.

As time went on, Ashley had many difficult situations; bleeding episodes necessitating many transfusions, side effects from medications involving three vertebral compression fractures, a foot fracture, acute kidney failure, and hospitalizations. Ashley's doctor was continually supportive in the hospital.

It was not long before the Appells discovered that their biggest hurdle was "school health services." When Ashley was denied access into the school district due to "medical fragility" and "potential liability," her doctor, a pediatric gastroenterologist, was Donna and Ashley's "pivotal" physician; he bridged the school and hospital systems. He established an emergency protocol for her school nurses and the local community hospital's emergency department. He documented the first-line medication and dosage used and listed the interventions needed to stabilize her until she could be transported to hospital or his office. Everyone was content with the support they received, and Ashley entered a school that was well prepared. Presently, she is thriving beautifully in eighth grade, and her physician continues to be by the Appells' side.

Donna realized the value of a relationship with a pivotal physician in her family's life.

The Support of Similarly Situated Parents

Maggie Hoffman gave birth to premature twins born at twenty-seven weeks. Jacob and Molly spent their first four and a half months in the neonatal intensive care unit with machines breathing for them and tubes feeding them. Maggie felt isolated as she heard her contemporaries discuss their

Mommy-and-Me programs and ached for that priceless feeling of the endless possibilities that should have been available to her perfect bundles.

The memories of her first year "at home" are a collage of airline flights for eye surgeries, stomach surgeries, and a legion of therapists, educators, and doctors. By fifteen months life had stabilized somewhat: Molly was fed intravenously through her broviac catheter, blind, in supportive seating, developmentally disabled, and showing an impressive array of seizure activity. Jacob had his own problems. If he were placed on a blanket outside, he would *feel* each blade of grass stabbing him. Sensations assaulted him. Little did Maggie know that his feeding disorder was due not only to his cerebral palsy but also to pervasive developmental disorder (PDD).

The twins turned two, a new baby was born, and Maggie's marriage dissolved. The family's private medical insurer went out of business, and Maggie became aware that she lived in the only county in the state without a Care-at-Home waiver program (New York State's medical assistance version of the Katie Beckett Waiver, which provides Medicaid eligibility for in-home care of children who would otherwise be placed in nursing homes). Appeals to government officials went unheeded. Finally, as it appeared that Molly's very sustenance was about to be cut off, a sympathetic and influential journalist wrote a column about their plight. Twenty-four hours later the county was signed on.

With all that was happening in her life, Maggie longed to socialize with peers. Were there any out there? In 1989 she created the New Survivors parent support group. Eventually, the credo of the New Survivors became clear: any family with a child with chronic illness has more in common than their child's particular diagnosis might suggest.

Molly died at the age of five and a half. Jacob, now a teenager and behaviorally challenged, attends a magnet school for children with autism. Jacob uses orthotics to support his gait, and he is a voracious reader. Maggie realized the importance of referrals to community resources and the value of parent-to-parent supports.

Focusing on Quality of Life

Nancy Speller's son John James (JJ), born in 1990, suffers from a neurotransmitter disease, an inborn error of metabolism that causes severe central nervous system damage. JJ's inability to metabolize Dopamine efficiently caused him gradually to lose his motor skills at a year old. Nancy was anguished watching her child deteriorate before her eyes and felt helpless to do anything for him. Today JJ is a flaccid quadriplegic and is dependent in all areas of daily living. Over the last few years JJ has also developed a severe movement disorder, which causes periods of intractable bilateral ballismus (involuntary movements). Like most children with chronic illness or disabilities, JJ has spent a large portion of his life in the hospital, visiting doctors and interacting with a multitude of health care professionals.

When JJ first became ill, Nancy diligently and aggressively pursued doctors, researchers, and anyone who was interested. She wanted to cure her son. Nancy believed if she looked hard enough, she would find the person with that miracle drug. There came a time in JJ's life, however, when Nancy needed to put aside his illness and disabilities and focus on finding her once happy child. She became extremely creative, finding new ways for him to play, to laugh, and to feel wonderful about himself. Then came a new, even more exasperating challenge: rallying the medical professionals to see past his illness and start focusing on how they could improve JJ's quality of life. Often Nancy would stand at JJ's bedside reminding doctors that he understood what was being said. Nancy would tire just from the effort it took ensuring that JJ's respect and dignity were being supported by the medical staff.

As a registered nurse, Nancy knew that chronic illness can be extremely frustrating for the professional. Medical education focuses on diseases and treatments; the goal is to make the patient better. What do you do, then, when you have no treatment and the outcome is not a good one? Nancy realized the value of promoting quality of life for the child and the family.

Three Tenets as the Foundation of Care

Even though each of us had a special situation to deal with, each of us quickly realized that our ardent concerns were shared issues. Speaking about these three necessary ingredients for a successful life in the community became our mission. We strongly believe that the following three tenets must form the foundation for care of an individual with chronic needs. Parents of children will special needs must be able to:

- partner with a pivotal physician;
- link to local and national resources; and
- promote quality of life.

Examining our lives and the lives of so many of our friends in similar circumstances, we saw that our children are "new survivors." With advances in medicine, pharmacology, and technology and the dawn of genetic testing, we are a new population of families with children with chronic illness and disabilities. Changes in health care insurance coverage often mean earlier discharge from a hospital, which creates greater care needs at home and in the community. Medical education needs to bridge the gap to support the lives outside of an acute care setting. An opportunity arose for us to formalize our vision and create a chronic care curriculum.

Project DOCC: A Chronic Care Curriculum

We were invited to pilot our curriculum as part of the pediatric residency training program at North Shore University Hospital, Manhasset, New York. Surrounded by Disney products, our spark came from the song "Colors of the Wind" in *Pocahontas:* "But if you walk the footsteps of a stranger, you'll learn things you never knew, you never knew." This theme so aptly describes the method of our program, by showing physicians how vital they are to our day-to-day lives.

Project DOCC (Delivery of Chronic Care) is a teaching program designed to incorporate all aspects and issues involved with the health care and education of children with chronic illness. It is a community-based program advocating for family-centered care and provides the tools and methodology for its implementation.

We believed that, if we reached doctors during their training years, family-centered delivery of chronic care would become automatic to their practice. Project DOCC is taught by parents. Parents are the basic foundation of a child's life and are well placed as teachers by virtue of their comprehensive role. They arrange for their child's medical care and educational life and provide financial security. Parents involve the child with his or her siblings and extended family and promote socialization and spirituality within their community. Parents participating in our program are required to complete a train-the-trainer session using our manuals, videos, and slides. Parents become faculty when they are able to teach Project DOCC core philosophies.

We focus on:

- the impact caused by chronic illness plus disability, not any specific disease or diagnosis;
- the family, not just the individual;
- speaking with one voice, advocating for one another about our universal issues—medical, financial, educational/career, social, spiritual;
- teaching, by positive example, to identify as models physicians and other professionals whose actions and caring have enhanced lives.

With these trained parent teachers, Project DOCC prepares, rehearses, and presents our five-hour, three-component curriculum. The first component is a Grand Rounds Panel Presentation. It is a moderated panel using personal stories and slides to illuminate the impact of chronicity on home and community life. One of the questions posed by a parent moderator to the panelists asks them to describe their transition from an acute situation in an otherwise "normal" life to a lifestyle filled with chronic care issues. One parent answers, "I realized that we had become *chronic* when my daughter had grown out of the largest size diaper Pampers sold." Another mother describes a morning, sipping coffee in her kitchen, a week after her son was discharged from a lengthy hospital stay: "I placed all of the doctors' business cards out in front of me at the table and was overwhelmed at the amount of follow-up appointments I'd have to make with all of these sub-specialists. It was at that moment that I understood chronicity." Each story builds on the next to create a total picture of our complex population.

The second component is a structured Home Visit, taught by two parent teachers. The first parent guides the resident through his or her home and describes "a-day-in-the-life." The second parent provides a global view by interjecting stories of other families' experiences. The subjective (Parent 1) and objective (Parent 2) views help to keep a pediatric resident focused on the impact on families rather than the particulars of any one child's profile.

The last component is the Parent Interview. This chronic illness history (questionnaire) is a discussion between the resident and a third parent teacher. The interview allows residents to ask intimate questions, delving into issues such as the rights of parents to determine care plans, training on new treatments and home equipment, limits of treatment, and Do Not Resuscitate orders. At the end of the interview residents are provided with a list of national and regional resources as well as some time to discuss related current events.

The overall design of the curriculum is to present Grand Rounds as an introduction of our new population; the Home Visit is a snapshot of a day in our lives; and the Parent Interview (using the Chronic Illness History) is a look into the family's journey. Success in our local hospital bought us an invitation to present our Grand Rounds Panel at a national conference. Unable to afford transportation for all five parent teachers, we asked the conference host to help us recruit panelists from the list of conference attendees. We were joined by parents from New Mexico, Texas, and Missouri; our presentation was seamless. As we suspected, families from around the country have the same issues. We were urged to "go national."

Project DOCC was implemented at four medical centers to test portability and the project's ability to be replicated. We supplied the materials (manuals, videos, and slides) free of charge, at the end of a two-day training, to teams of families who had partnered with a medical center. Each site had to agree to mandate each resident's participation. Informal evaluations seemed to support our theses: parent teachers felt empowered, residents were motivated, and directors of residency training saw value in the program.

Finances have been a real stumbling block for Project DOCC. We reject the idea of selling the curriculum to individual medical centers. Project DOCC is a grassroots, family-driven program. Since we are not direct-service providers, it has been hard to attract individual donors. Grant-making foundations such as the United Hospital Fund have been Project DOCC's major supporters.

We have been training residents since 1994. Project DOCC is currently in more than twenty medical centers coast to coast and two in Australia. Additionally, Project DOCC is piloting a curriculum for older adults and their family caregivers.

Conclusion

Our vision is to see the concepts of chronic care taught to all medical students and residents. We continue our mission to promote an understanding of the issues involved in caring for a family living with special health care needs regardless of age, diagnosis, or prognosis; to put the family at the center of the health care system. We are grateful to all those who have given us the opportunity to make our children's lives count.

CHAPTER ELEVEN

Changing Institutional Culture

Turning Adversaries into Partners

Judah L. Ronch

When cultures of caregiving come into contact, conflict often results. "Consumers," that is, patients and family members, and "providers," health care professionals and paraprofessionals, all too frequently disagree (Levine and Zuckerman 1999; also Levine and Murray, in Chapter 1 of this volume). Because conflict narratives (experienced firsthand or recounted as stories after they unfold) are built upon the foundation of their respective cultural values and behavioral expectations, they represent and reinforce the belief systems of each side (Bruner 2002.)

These conflicts also represent more than a clash between health care consumers and providers. On a more fundamental level there is a gap between the cultural assumptions that characterize how health care and family systems operate as social institutions (Harrington 2000.) For example, the health care institution is organized and operated according to traditional hierarchic, power-oriented, "masculine" relationship models (O'Toole 1996), while the family, at least in its common American incarnation, typically operates according to more collaborative and nonhierarchical, "feminine" organizational principles (John-Steiner 2000; Helgesen 1995; Gilligan 1993.) When these incompatible organizational principles meet in the hospital, nursing home, or other health care setting, conflict often breaks out.

The essential competition is over control of how care will be provided, with a corollary conflict over what actions, and by whom, constitute good care. As a result, employees in the health care setting are expected to, and usually do, line up with their peers and "teammates" and conform to existing norms of mutual support and worker role identity. They thus constitute the "solution team" (Eron and Lund 2003), seeing themselves as best suited to address the challenge of illness or trauma. To care providers, the patient and his or her family, on the other hand, represent the adversary, or the "problem team."

This alignment of participants as adversaries creates the battleground for conflict and competition as the "solution team" seeks to assert its dominance and impose its own cultural values. Those who represent or embody competing cultural systems of care are seen as obstacles to their success (Levine and Zuckerman 1999.) This alignment into competing teams can create significant stress among health care professionals when their own relatives become patients, since they are torn between their motivations to act primarily as family members, in spite of their immersion in and familiarity with their usual roles as health care providers (see Chapter 9, by Jeffrey Blustein, in this volume).

The operative metaphor is *conflict as war,* in which there must a winner and a loser. There is, however, an alternate view of conflict—*conflict as opportunity or journey* (Cloke and Goldsmith 2000). This alternate perspective sees conflict as a natural outgrowth of the diversity in knowledge, culture, technical expertise, values, and the specialized roles played by providers and patients/families. It assumes that opponents can achieve more of their mutual goals when they are allies rather than enemies. The parties perceived as adversaries in the war scenario are transformed in the "opportunity and journey" scenarios into an essential source of help. The value of conflict, in this view, is that it allows the divergent cultural frames and their underlying values, diverse sources of information and knowledge, and individual perceptions of the health event to inform the process and expand possibilities for problem solving. Here everyone is on the solution team.

The stakeholders become *conflict resolution partners* (Weeks 1992) who, because they are now able to collaborate, achieve better outcomes than each could alone. As this is taking place, their relationship improves as a result of sharing the experience of working on the problem together. Their mutual focus increases the likelihood of turning a vicious cycle into a virtuous one as well as lowering stress and anger levels for all involved. Perhaps this alternative view of conflict's most valuable contribution is that it requires partners in conflict resolution to see how values held by the other partners are not barriers to the exercise of "positive power," that is, power that strengthens the helpful contribution of others.

From another perspective, when conflict is seen as an opportunity or journey rather than as a war, a new emphasis on relationship building can supplant a zero-sum, "win-lose" approach. Emphasis on the "right way" to provide care deters relationship building among all participants and denies the reality that all are entering a relationship of unknown duration due to a mutual need. In that relationship each has a contribution, but not the exclusive role, in determining the quality of care.

In an attempt to apply the "conflict as opportunity" model to the traditional dimensions of conflict, I have selected several major issues around which friction typically arises between the solution team and the problem team. Moreover, I have proposed briefly how an approach using a model such as the conflict resolution partnership might apply. While a more thorough review of conflict resolution models and the valuable skills they represent is beyond the scope of this chapter, I hope to show the value of an institutional culture of conflict resolution partnership. Through easily learned skills, such an alternative to conflict as war could be of practical help in improving the experience of both providers and consumers in the health care system (see, e.g., Weeks 1992; Cloke and Goldsmith 2000; Levine 1998; McClure 2000.)

The five key principles of this new pathway are:

1. Every stakeholder has expertise about something but not about everything.
2. Everyone in the institutional setting has a family (for better or worse).
3. Everyone needs to feel important, needed, useful, and successful.
4. All people are at their best when they behave in accordance with their positive aspirations and views of themselves.

5. Everyone wants to be informed as completely as possible about the situation: ignorance breeds anxiety, fear, and anger and fuels the conflict cycle.

Different Kinds of Expertise

Principle 1. Every stakeholder has expertise about something but not about everything.

In its simplest formulation conflict often arises over the answer to the question: "Does the person have the illness, or does the illness have the person?"

Health care providers have been trained to be and to see themselves as experts about illnesses; they have a special, valuable view based on empiricism and scientific methods. Among patients with the same health problem, distinguishing characteristics such as personality, family dynamics, and cultural and sociodemographic factors are often subordinated or not factored into the care process. Sometimes they are seen (if at all) as nuisance, not substance (Levine and Zuckerman 1999). Except for information included in the medical history, the patient is viewed as if he or she appeared de novo at the health care setting. In hospitals even critical information such as dementia is not usually included in the medical chart of patients admitted for other reasons because only the primary diagnosis—the trigger for reimbursement—matters. In this worldview the patient is at risk of being treated as a mere vessel containing the illness.

Family members and the patient, on the other hand, are and see themselves as experts about the person, if not the illness. For them the illness has occurred in the context of the ongoing life experience of the person(s) involved. The change in health status is not an isolated event, and they tend to respond according to its impact on their daily lives as viewed through their particular cultural, familial, and socioeconomic lenses. This conflict of views reflects the difference between the culture of health care professionals and the culture of families about whether an illness or other health condition is seen as passively hosted (the illness has the patient) or actively experienced (the patient has the illness). That is, health care professionals might see the illness, or at least their role in it, as biographically neutral, while to the family it is part of their ongoing life story (or narrative). If an illness is actively experienced, then it is critical for the practitioner to identify the impact of the illness, the concomitant alterations on view(s) of self, and how the illness influences body and mind. The interrelated physical and psychological responses to the illness and how these will influence the eventual adaptation or recovery by the patient and family members (including all non–biologically related significant others) are significant data for the practitioner to consider in treatment planning.

Sacks addressed the unity of patient and illness when he wrote of what it means to be ill: "It must be said from the outset," Sacks wrote, "that a disease is never a mere loss or excess—that there is *always* a reaction, on the part of the affected organism or individual, to preserve, to restore, to replace, to compensate for, and to preserve its identity, however strange the means may be" (1985, 4). His advice to practitioners may be read as a caution to clinicians that patients' behaviors aimed at "self-preservation" during an illness are an integral part of the illness' clinical presentation and that to ignore these blinds us to the true nature of the illness and its optimal treatment for that person.

The two perspectives—the patient as passive vessel or active participant in the illness—come into conflict because they differ explicitly with regard to whose expertise is primary and whose frame of reference will characterize the future interactions of all stakeholders. They also diverge over the importance of individual differences among patients and families and how they might be engaged to improve outcomes and promote wellness.

No illness, real or imagined, arrives at the institution's threshold for health care without a person (the patient). So, it would seem desirable to identify common ground where these cultural views might meet. The illusion that the person and illness are separable works against a collaborative resolution of conflict because it requires one or the other stakeholder to abandon central values and beliefs for the care process to proceed. This conflict results when ego-centered goals have priority over problem-centered ones. In Sacks's sense all of those affected by the illness—patient, family member, and paid caregiver—need to experience themselves, and need to be seen by the other stakeholders, as helpful or expert about what they know best. The family and patient know the patient with the illness; the professionals know the illness affecting the patient. Conflict resolution that takes advantage of what both know and how both cultures add knowledge that can work in complementary ways will lead to optimal outcomes for the patient and maximal self-esteem for caregivers.

Providers as Family and as "Family"

Principle 2. Everyone in the institutional setting has a family (for better or worse).

How the patient's and family's experience of illness informs the nature of care (Cotrell and Schulz 1993) and whether they respond by actively participating in the care process and play a significant role in promoting positive outcomes, motivating health-relevant behaviors, and improving survival rates (Salovey, Rothman, Detweiler, and Steward 2000). Because nearly all patients and staff in institutional health care settings have families, the impact of their family membership cannot be ignored. Past and present family relationships have been influenced by, and continue to influence, both the family of origin (the most critical contextual influence on psychosocial development) and current family systems.

Both these sets of influences accompany the patient when he or she is admitted into any health care setting. It has long been an axiom of family therapy that any change in one family member stimulates changes in the entire system and everyone in it (Ackerman 1958). Therefore, an illness or any other change in functional status influences the patient and the family system and all its members. Relationships may change; alliances among relatives may be created and recreated; and the psychological health of the family system may be vulnerable as the family members contend with the new condition.

Patients and family members do not necessarily view the illness or its impact in the same way merely because they are kin. The family is not necessarily a single-minded unit (see Chapter 9 by Blustein, in this volume). Each member may experience the same illness differently and may hold divergent and often conflicting ideas about what should be done for, with, and to the patient. Patients and family members, like all stakeholders, are actually members of a family system composed of many subsystems (e.g., sibling, spousal, parental), which accompany them through the door of the institutional setting. While each of these systems and subsystems may differ in its dynamics, strengths, and tolerance to the stresses created by an illness, all these variables will influence what practitioners may observe in the behavior of each family member and what family members see in one another. This complex, composite picture of family dynamics inside and outside the institution constitutes the "family response" to the illness.

Staff members also bring the essence of their own family experiences to work with them. Their family dynamics and family history will, in turn, color their reactions to patients and their families (in a process called "appraisal" if it is conscious and "countertransference" if it is operating on the unconscious level) and create an additional dynamic contribution to the entire domain of familial influence in the institutional setting. While all the stakeholders do not usually acknowledge this kind of complex interaction of multiple family dynamics, it is a powerful influence on relationships and individual stakeholder behavior, especially in those most intimately and directly involved with the illness event.

That said, a person's identity within the family systems and subsystems (functional or dysfunctional as they may be at any given time) is most often stronger and more deeply embedded in the sense of self than is his or her identity as a patient or institutional resident. Health care professionals often act as though a person with an illness, and their family members, is required to suspend or subordinate these relationships or risk not being seen as a "good patient." If patient and family members hold a view that departs from institutional culture and request or demand that the culture of the institution adapt to personal or family needs, the family/patient constellation is likely to be labeled as "resistant." They are at risk of being "punished" for their uncooperative behavior if practitioners categorize them as problem patients or label them "dysfunctional" families (Levine and Zuckerman 1999). Family members so labeled are at risk of being treated as threats to the institutional system. In turn, families may escalate the crisis or retreat and fail to inform staff adequately about vital patient information or advocate sufficiently for their family members.

"Family feuds" over control are ultimately "problem-maintaining solutions" (Eron and Lund 1996), since without meaning to they perpetuate the very problem—lack of family cooperation—which they have been trying to solve. But, above all, they may lead to suboptimal outcomes, anger, and the conscious or unconscious scapegoating of vulnerable institutional patients whose family members are considered a problem. Staff begin to feel "damned if they do and damned if they don't" and respond with passivity and distance, if not with overt hostility poorly disguised as artificial politeness or neglect. This is not the way most staff members prefer to behave, but it is an inevitable and unfortunate component of a culturally sanctioned tendency to view institutional admission as the occasion for family members to subordinate all family ties for the duration of the patient's stay (or until discharge is imminent) and turn all caregiving and related decision making over to the staff.

Conflicts arise when sibling rivalry–like disputes arise under these conditions; conflict breaks out over who will care for the patient most expertly and, in so doing, enhance his or her own self-esteem. Since high stress levels tend to produce regression and defensiveness (Maslow 1998), participants in such scenarios are unable to collaborate very well. The solution may emerge when each "rival" is able to see the other's intentions as valid and important but rooted in his or her respective different cultural or family systems. A potential collaborative partnership resolution would recognize that the resident has not divorced his or her family any more than did the staff members divorce theirs when they came to work that day and that each rival is in actuality a member of a temporary blended family.

In this newly constituted family system each member has the opportunity to confirm his or her preferred view by contributing knowledge to the task of preserving the individuality of the patient during the illness (Eron and Lund 1996). Most families do not "let go" of patients in toto at the time of institutional admission but, rather, initiate an individualized pattern of transition in which some aspects of care are continued and others are handed over to paid caregivers (Zarit and Whitlatch 1992). Each family has a somewhat different pattern and requires a period of adjustment and a negotiated transition. Each stakeholder—patient, family, and care provider—can be helped to achieve optimal self-esteem and a feeling of competence. In a "win-win" scenario all participants collaborate in deciding how each can continue to do what he or she does best in this new "family relationship" and provide the best possible care for the patient.

Emphasizing Success

Principle 3. Everyone needs to feel important, needed, useful, and successful.

Adversarial stances tend to occur when providers fail to appreciate how disturbing it may be to the patient and family members to need medical help. The act of introducing a health care professional—even when the patient acknowledges the need—may signal that the patient or family might perceive themselves, or fear being seen by others, as somehow inadequate. Even if the need for help is not questioned, the situation may prompt anxiety, sadness, disappointment, lethargy, depression, resignation (passive compliance), anger, resistance, and other negative emotional states (Eron and Lund 1996). Family members or patients may construe the need for professional caregiving as a sign that their efforts have failed and that the community or other family members will see them as not having been sufficiently dedicated to the person's care. They might fear that they will be viewed as not having done right by the patient.

Professional health care providers, conditioned to thinking of themselves as being helpful, well-trained, and even heroic, are prone to interpret patient and family responses such as resistance, passivity, or anger as signs of individual or family pathology. They may plan their care strategy based on these often incorrect and unyielding assessments. A patient and family who do not share dominant cultural frames with paid health providers are more likely to face multiple jeopardy and be subject to having their behavior framed in pathologizing terms by facility staff when they express differences or grievances with the institutional culture. The result is that the patient and family are more likely to be treated in what M. Buber (1970) terms the "I-it" relationship (person as object), rather than to be met as people within an "I-thou" relationship of equal human beings.

Some sources of multiple jeopardy which may lead to misattribution of patients' and families' responses to helpers in contemporary health care settings, including the home, are:

- the impact of illness on physical and functional status;
- sexism, homophobia, and gender stereotypes;
- age and the negative effects of ageism;
- racial and ethnic differences from health providers;
- socioeconomic status;
- cognitive impairment, real or presumed, which leads providers to interact with patients or families as though they have limited intelligence and faulty judgment;
- nonnative speech patterns or poor communication skills in the language of the dominant culture, which may lead to the assumptions of limited intelligence or poor cognition;
- impaired hearing or vision;
- chronic illness;
- physical handicap;

- co-morbid psychiatric illness, whether chronic or acute; and
- role of family members (e.g., spouse, offspring, significant other) and the impact of these sources of jeopardy on how the family member is viewed by paid care providers.

If providers engage in adversarial behavior, the family and patient will become stuck attempting to satisfy their more basic safety or defensive needs (Maslow 1998) and will be less available to play a useful role as partners in health care. If any stakeholder feels threatened, unimportant, anonymous, expendable, or disrespected, these reactions will stimulate conflict and competition over whose needs will be met. This conflict may become the dominant agenda for the interactions between professional caregivers and family members and prevent their collaboration about more important issues, such as what is likely to be of most value in helping the patient/family system and how collaboration may help staff produce better clinical results.

Accentuating the Positive

Principle 4. All people are at their best when they behave in accordance with their positive aspirations and views of themselves.
Devaluing and discounting patients' and family members' positive traits imposes and reinforces their disempowered, subordinate status. Reasonable requests to share power through assertiveness, voicing their preferences, or indicating choices for themselves or the patient are all too apt to be labeled aggressiveness, "inappropriate behavior," resistance, "oppositionalism," and other jargon for not cooperating with the "authorities." These devices are culturally approved ways to wrap staff feelings in pseudoscientific stigmatizing labels that really mean: "I don't like your attitude" and "You have no right to demand to be treated as an equal because I am an expert in health care and therefore in this setting am better than you."

Persons who have been labeled by the "experts" (the paid care providers) with diagnostic labels or professional insider jargon are as a result seen as occupying socially devalued roles (Wolfensberger 1985.) As a consequence, they are believed to be motivated by undesirable (primitive, pathological) impulses, naïveté, or ignorance. All of their problematic behaviors come to be attributed to the "diagnosis" (formal or informal), rather than to legitimate desires for self-affirmation or a universal need to support their self-esteem when faced with a loss of power and marginalization.

It is easy for providers to slip into this mind-set when, for example, they interact with patients and family members of another culture or those who are older, anxious, and feeling vulnerable. This further aggravates the potentially disturbing effects of needing help and promotes dissonant behavior at the time when collaboration to engage the strengths of the family and patient are most needed.

Demands that the family or patient accept the validity of others' view of them by acting as others see them tend to generate more of the stigmatized behavior. For example, family members may respond to such treatment with belligerence, apathy, depression, negativism, or resistance (Eron and Lund 1996). They may withdraw from taking responsibility for things well within their capability. In their attempts to be helpful, institutional staff frequently require patients and family members to agree with their (professional and more expert) view of the problem so that all the stakeholders may begin to "act like a team." This demand unfortunately only serves to increase the rigidity of the patient's and family's position and reduces the likelihood of their being able to mobilize their team skills. This becomes a classic problem-maintaining solution and prevents a true team from being constituted among the stakeholders. A problem-solving partnership requires understanding that conflict resolution involves assessing how all participants in the conflict view themselves, their conflict partners, the conflict, and the relationship before attempting a solution. Teams must develop norms of activity, generate potential solutions in an atmosphere of mutual respect, and work together on common problems in real time.

Communication Strategies

Principle 5. Everyone wants to be informed as completely as possible about the situation: ignorance breeds anxiety, fear, and anger and fuels the conflict cycle.

Clashes of culture between patients family members and providers are exacerbated by the degree of institutional control (Goffman 1961; Bennett 1963) and by the way in which resulting cultural lore generates and maintains the various explanations of other peoples' behavior. This effect is seen most clearly in staff explanations or understanding about how patients (Gubrium 1975), family members, and other outsiders act. Care providers skillfully speak the professional jargon and describe people's behavior in the language of the dominant culture in the institution (e.g., diagnostic and technical terms). Doing so legitimizes their very presence and their repertoire of interventions. But it also frequently perpetuates the very problem behavior they object to (Wolfensberger 1985).

Families also bring their own cultural lore as a frame of reference for understanding what they see in providers' behavior. They may generate explanations of staff behavior based on their particular understanding of institutional lore or as a result of family experiences, myths, or relatives' attributions (accurate or not) about staff behavior ("The nurses ignore the patients; the doctors are never available.") Although the possibilities of mis-attribution and misunderstanding are many, the powerful influence of the institution on the behavior of all stakeholders is seen in findings that student volunteers playing the role of nursing home residents begin to manifest "un-desirable" institutional behaviors in *as little as forty-eight hours* (Wigdor, Nelson, and Hickerson 1977).

Interpersonal communication issues, and the way in which information is transmitted in the institution constitute another major barrier to conflict resolution using conflict resolution partnerships. In most traditional health care settings communication rules are characterized by a hierarchical, "top-down" flow of information and strict rules governing access to patient information. There is a culturally maintained division among higher-status (professional) and lower-status (para- or nonprofessional) care providers about who may be privy to what information, what are the acceptable uses of information, and who may appropriately use technical terms (see Diamond 1992.)

Socially marked rules of communication and the accompanying social sanctions for breaking them within institutions are largely defined by, and define, social class membership. This is reflected in settings where only the high-status experts are allowed to use the jargon and technical terminology whose use denotes intelligence and experience. The higher-ups in the institutional hierarchy are perceived to possess the more valuable information, and their use of language reinforces that perception. In health care staff members' use of sophisticated medical terminology or code words and abbreviations is in one sense an exercise of power. Lower-status, less-empowered people, such as nonmedical personnel or families who try to speak the higher-status code or gain access to some types of information, may be seen as violators of the cultural rules and reminded of their proper place. These hierarchical, exclusive communication patterns unfortunately function as another disincentive for teamwork among the stakeholders, despite the current popularity of advertising the team approach as a self-designated badge of professionalism in many institutions.

In contemporary institutional cultures it is all too often deemed necessary that the solution team communicate with the problem team only to advance the solution team's agenda. The "white coat barrier" is used to seal off extensive conversations about the patient and his or her care from the problem team and its members' competing view of things. The barrier is rationalized and perpetuated by traditional institutional care procedures that fit the prevailing culturally supported perception that assertive care recipients and their family members, and staff members who align with their views, are only sources of communicative dissonance.

Conflict resolution partnership activity may begin when staff members are able to attribute the desires of family and self-assertive patients to be in the communication loop as attempts at problem solving rather than problem creating. In other words, the attempts of the family and patient to be involved in determining the nature of care are in line with their view of themselves as being caring, autonomous, capable, and informed. This is so even if their attempts are unusual in the context of the institutional culture. Such a transition is especially critical when we remember providers' tendency to see such attempts at inclusion as evidence of pathology, which in turn often creates or exacerbates the very behavior they find objectionable and reinforces the "us versus them" relationship.

The majority of patients and family members probably did not wake up on any given day and decide to be a pain in the neck for the practitioners. Nevertheless, care providers frequently respond to them as though what lies behind their attempts to be on the solution team is primarily a conscious and malevolent desire to challenge or undermine the medical or technical expertise of the providers and to make them feel bad. Their motivation is probably better understood as rooted in their desire to lower their anxiety, reduce their fear, and contribute their valid expertise about the life and/or "experience of the illness" of the patient and themselves. But they cannot contribute in a meaningful way if they are met with hostility, exclusion, or related threats.

Conclusion

Because the illness is in some sense a crisis for each family which threatens to disrupt its narrative significantly and redefine its interpersonal equilibrium (such as by creating or intensifying the dependency of one member on another) or its integrity (by the possibility of the death of a family member), the increasingly dominant role played by emotional, subjective modes of interacting with others is natural in such crises. The family and patient might look inward toward their core values even more than before for guidance and comfort. Turning inward for moral and ethical guidance for personal actions is especially likely for family members as they confront the emotional impacts of an illness in the family and the threats attendant to entering the physical, social, psychological, and other manifestations of an unfamiliar culture (uniforms, impersonal environments, strict rules of access to places such as the intensive care unit and to people such as the physician, head nurse, or administrator) as well as the experience of loss of control over their lives and their family dynamics which the institutional culture demands.

During an illness the predominantly subjective imperatives of intimacy, commitment, and caring which govern family culture (see intro. by Levine and Murray, in this volume) are easily thrown into conflict with the objectivist, rational, techno-scientific aspects of procedures and practices that typify modern health care institutions. These environments are organized around procedures that rely on the most objective, emotionally detached evaluation by practitioners of the data about a patient's medical status generated to a large degree by the most advanced (and often anxiety-producing and mysterious) technology available. The information derived from the various high-tech, low-touch assessments may be treated and discussed almost as if it had an existence beyond the corporeal boundaries of the patient. The practitioner's or care provider's emotions are filtered out or cleansed from the clinical analyses and treatment decisions as much as possible.

These two vastly different mind-sets of the family and the health care institution, which represent the essence of what permits each respective culture to thrive in its own environment, come into conflict when practitioners and patients and their family members struggle over which ethos will prevail and thus provide the moral, logical framework for conversations about care in the institution. Because practitioners hold the power in institutions, the patient/family constellation constantly confronts imperatives in the institution which are quite at odds with what has historically bound them together. In addition to the strain the illness has created in the family, relatives must absorb the additional stress of turning over the care of one of their own to representatives of a culture whose values and practices are alien to them. Perhaps in their view it is also a threat to the well-being of their family member if he or she is "separated" from them and the benefit of the nurturing embrace of their relationship.

When family members attempt to follow through on their values and their subjective, unconditional moral injunctions in the objectivist health care setting, they may experience resistance from providers. If a family yields, it may then encounter the stress of a guilt-inducing and depressing double-bind situation for having failed to provide for its relative according to the dictates of the family value structure. Its options consist of having to abandon its culturally appropriate role (i.e., surrendering control) in order to obtain medical care or to follow the injunction and perhaps sacrifice access to what modern science, embedded in the context of the institutional culture of care, could potentially provide to make the family member well.

One solution to this conflict lies in creating a culture through a collaborative process which uses the strengths of both subjective and objective positions. My experience has been that health care providers, especially those in paraprofessional positions and those managers who are empathic practitioners, have emotional sensitivity to their own feelings generated by what they do and empathy for the patients' and family member's experiences. Family members and patients are capable of honoring their obligations to one another and to themselves and are willing to collaborate with practitioners if their strengths—emotional loyalty, assuming the caregiving responsibility, representing the interests of the patient's quality of life, love, and concern even at great sacrifice to one's own well-being, and a shared sense of history with the patient—are acknowledged and valued.

REFERENCES

Ackerman, N. (1958). *The Psychodynamics of Family Life*. New York: Basic Books.
Bennett, R. (1963). "The Meaning of Institutional Life." *Gerontologist* 3:117–25.
Bruner, J. S. (2002). *Making Stories*. New York: Farrar, Straus and Giroux.
Buber, M. (1970). *I and Thou*. New York: Charles Scribner and Sons.

Cloke, K. and J. Goldsmith. (2000). *Resolving Conflicts at Work.* San Francisco: Jossey-Bass.

Cotrell, V., and R. Schulz, (1993). "The Perspective of the Patient with Alzheimer's Disease: A Dimension of Dementia Research." *Gerontologist* 33:205–11.

Diamond, T. (1992). *Making Gray Gold.* Chicago: University of Chicago Press.

Eron, J., and T. Lund. (1996). *Narrative Solutions in Brief Therapy.* New York: Guilford Press.

———. (2003). "The Narrative Solutions Approach: Bringing Out the Best in People as They Age." In *Mental Wellness in Aging: Strengths-based Approaches,* ed. J. Ronch and J. Goldfield, 273–98. Baltimore: Health Professions Press.

Gilligan, C. (1993). *In a Different Voice.* Cambridge, Mass.: Harvard University Press.

Goffman, E. (1961). *Asylums: Essays on the Social Situation of Mental Patients and Other Inmates.* Garden City, N.Y.: Anchor Books.

Gubrium, J. (1975) *Living and Dying in Murray Manor.* New York: St. Martin's Press.

Harrington, M. (2000). *Care and Equality.* New York: Routledge.

Helgesen, S. (1990). *The Female Advantage: Women's Ways of Leadership.* New York: Currency Doubleday.

John-Steiner, V. (2000). *Creative Collaboration.* New York: Oxford University Press.

Levine, C. (2003). "Family Caregivers, Health Care Professionals and Policy Makers: The Diverse Cultures of Long-Term Care." In *Culture Change in Long-Term Care,* Ed. A. S. Weiner and J. Ronch. Binghamton, N.Y.: Hayworth Press.

Levine, C., and C. Zuckerman. (1999). "The Trouble with Families." *Annals of Internal Medicine* 130:148–52.

Maslow, A. (1998). *Maslow on Management.* New York: John Wiley.

McClure, L. (2000). *Anger and Conflict in the Workplace.* Manassas Park, Va.: Impact Publishers.

O'Toole, J. (1996). *Leading Change.* New York: Ballantine Books.

Sacks, O. (1985). *The Man Who Mistook His Wife for a Hat.* New York: Summit Books.

Salovey, P., A. Rothman, J. Detweiler, and W. Steward. (2000). "Emotional States and Physical Health." *American Psychologist* 55:1.

Weeks. D. (1992). *The Eight Essential Steps to Conflict Resolution* New York: Jeremy P. Tarcher Putnam.

Wigdor, R. N., J. Nelson, and E. Hickerson. (1977, Nov. 18–22). "The Behavioral Comparison of a Real vs. Mock Nursing Home." Presented at the annual meeting of the Gerontological Society, San Francisco.

Wolfensberger, W. (1985). "An Overview of Social Role Valorization and Some Reflections on Elderly Mentally Retarded Persons." In *Aging and Developmental Disabilities,* ed. M. Janicki and H. Wisniewski. Baltimore: Brooks.

Zarit, S., and C. J. Whitlatch. (1992). "Institutional Placement: Phases of Transition." *Gerontologist* 32:665–72.

Conclusion

Building on Common Ground

Carol Levine and Thomas H. Murray

When faced with a daunting challenge like bringing understanding and accommodation to disparate cultures, it is all too tempting to throw up one's
metaphorical hands in despair and move on. As the chapters in this volume
document, there is indeed a gap between the cultures of family caregiving and
the different health care professionals they encounter. But another theme in
the book is that there is also common ground on which to build.

Despite common misperceptions, cultures are not static constructs. They
do change, and often rapidly, when there are motivated change agents and a
rationale or external pressure that resonates within the culture. While the core
values of family relationships such as fidelity and a shared history remain constant, family structures and practices have undergone major changes, not just
in contemporary society but also throughout history. In health care, consider
the major change that occurred in a relatively short time as childbirth practices responded to parents' demands and became more humane and family
centered. A similar shift is under way in end-of-life care, although it has by no
means reached the mainstream. It is possible, though difficult, to bring about
a shift in organizational and provider cultures toward a system that is more

responsive to family caregivers; it is equally possible, but no less difficult, to give family caregivers a better understanding of and better tools to deal with the diverse professional and bureaucratic cultures of health care.

This concluding chapter brings together some of the suggestions and insights presented in the preceding chapters, and offers some additional ones as well, about ways that family caregivers, health care professionals, and others in the health care system can begin to adapt in ways that reflect a deeper understanding of their differences and, in so doing, help to bridge the culture gap. Equipped with these ideas, they will be better able to achieve their common goal—the best possible care for ill or disabled people and the best possible quality of life for both them and their caregivers. These suggestions are divided into three main areas: research, education and training, and policies and programs.

Research

Although there is a vast literature on family caregiving and an even more voluminous one on the attitudes and behaviors of health care professionals, very little of either literature addresses our thesis that family caregivers and health care professionals bring different priorities and assumptions to the care of an ill person. Much of the family caregiving literature ignores the care recipient's relationship to the health care system and portrays caregiving as primarily a supportive or difficult relationship between two people or at most within a family. Much of the medical or nursing literature that mentions families at all is limited to platitudes or portrays families as impediments to professionals' doing their jobs efficiently and authoritatively. There are, of course, exceptions, and many of the contributors to this volume, as well as others, have written eloquently about family issues.

Still, we believe strongly that much more research needs to be done. David Gould's chapter describes the results of one survey of family caregivers which began to examine the interaction of family caregivers with the health care system. This survey documented, first, that family caregivers take care not only of people who are old and frail but also people of all ages suffering from a number of chronic illnesses; 50 percent of the care recipients were hospitalized in the year preceding the survey. Second, family caregivers receive inadequate training about the medical aspects of care, including changing bandages, monitoring equipment, and managing medications. Often what little training they do get comes not from the professionals directly involved with the patient but from someone the caregiver knows or consults informally.

This survey was unusual in even asking about the medical aspects of family caregiving. Further studies should be conducted to provide more data to give a comprehensive picture of what caregivers actually do in this and other domains. Thus, as Gould points out, we need more precise measures to define and capture the full range and complexity of caregiver tasks beyond the commonly used Activities of Daily Living (ADL) and Instrumental Activities of Daily Living (IADL) measures (Levine 2004). Without this knowledge, health care professionals cannot respond intelligently and comprehensively to caregivers' needs. Furthermore, Gould recommends the development of better hospital discharge planning procedures to train family caregivers and to put in place appropriate home care services.

The chapters by Mathy Mezey, Sheila Rothman, and Rick Surpin and Eileen Hanley describe the evolution of relationships between family caregivers and home care providers such as nurses and home care aides. Although the survey results described by Gould showed that very few family caregivers had assistance from paid home care aides, caregivers who are employed, in particular, will increasingly turn to outside help. Understanding more about the dynamics of this relationship is crucial. While doctors and family caregivers often meet at critical decision-making times, nurses and home care aides are more likely to be involved in day-to-day care and management. Their interactions are no less important. Yet, as Surpin and Hanley point out, we know very little about what actually goes on within the home.

We need much more detailed and nuanced information about the impact of hospitalization and discharge on the family caregiver and his or her responsibilities, the interaction between family caregivers and representatives of the formal home care system such as home care agency administrators and workers, and what happens when formal home care ends. These transitions are key points in the caregiver "career." One such study is under way at the United Hospital Fund. Called "This Case Is Closed: How Family Caregivers Manage the Transition When Home Care Services Are Terminated," the study is following one hundred family caregivers of patients with stroke or traumatic brain injury for a year to investigate what caregivers do to substitute for paid care and how it affects them as well as patients' rehabilitation and quality of life. Another cohort of one hundred family caregivers will be interviewed retrospectively.

Jeffrey Blustein describes the situations in which health care professionals become family caregivers and find themselves as overwhelmed by the challenges as their lay counterparts. A large-scale study of nurses found that many are leaving the profession not just because of poor working conditions and low salaries but because they are also the family caregivers of elderly relatives and do not trust the system to provide adequate home care (Monahan and Hopkins 2002). Studies of health care professionals as family caregivers would give us more insights into how their disciplinary backgrounds influence their own family caregiving choices. These caregivers, with links to both cultures, can offer special insights and recommendations for better communication and practices.

Much of the work that has been done so far is quantitative; while there are clear advantages to such studies, we also need more qualitative work to provide the depth and diversity to the experiences of family caregivers and professionals as they encounter each other. We need to know more about professionals' attitudes, practices, and fears about loss of control which occurs in home care that influence their relationships with family caregivers and patients. The perspectives of all the participants is crucial—family members, physicians, nurses, professionals such as physical and speech therapists, and the invaluable home care aides. The shortage of home care workers is troubling now and ominous for the future. We need to know how to make this difficult job more attractive, and we suspect that, beyond the real problems of low wages and few benefits, a significant reason for the poor retention of workers is the uneasy relationships with families, patients, and agency personnel. We know nothing at all about the "gray market" in home care workers, that is, aides who are hired and paid privately. The gray market exists because new immigrants, concerned about regulations and bureaucracies, may not want to work for a certified home health agency. Family members hire them mainly because they cannot afford agency rates; some may also prefer to control the arrangements themselves. Sometimes this works well for both; sometimes it is exploitative for the worker and unsatisfactory for the patient and family.

We also know very little about the quality of care provided by family caregivers. Unless there are egregious instances of abuse or neglect, family care is outside the scope of any quality monitoring. Yet, if trained providers are not immune from error, it seems reasonable to assume that untrained and over-whelmed family members will from time to time make mistakes, no matter how good their intentions or how loving their care. One study of four hundred discharged hospital patients found that adverse events occurred at home in 19 percent, some of them serious enough to require rehospitalization (Forster et al. 2003). The authors concluded that nearly all the problems could have been prevented by better communication and discharge planning. At the same time it is unrealistic to hold family caregivers to the same level of technical proficiency as professionals. Before a serious discussion on quality in family care can take place, we need to know more about the reality.

In short, we need both quantitative studies and an ethnography of home care which describes the various cultures that exist within it and the structures and belief systems that both affect home care and are influenced by it.

Education and Training

If there is one recommendation on which all authors would likely agree, it is that education and training are essential for all those involved in providing or assisting family caregivers and for the caregivers themselves. Mezey, Surpin and Hanley, Judah Ronch, and Maggie Hoffman and Donna Jean Appell address this aspect directly; others do it indirectly.

Much of the needed education and training will be task oriented or aimed at problem solving. While a cultural divide as we have conceptualized it may not be the most visible aspect of education, it will play an important role in the language and tone of the presentations, the ways in which family care-givers and professionals are engaged in the sessions, and how well the teaching recognizes the many ways in which attitudes and behaviors reflect one's primary perspective, whether that is family or professional discipline. To give one example, caregivers in a series of United Hospital Fund focus groups consistently said that hospital professionals who tried to show them how to take care of their family member who was about to be discharged to home, whether that involved operating a machine or changing bandages or any other responsibility, failed to appreciate the emotional component. For the professional it was routine; family caregivers who hesitated or fumbled were seen as inept or unwilling to learn. For the family member it was learning to do something difficult or painful or embarrassing for the first time for someone they loved. A simple acknowledgment of that anxiety would have gone a long way toward helping family caregivers feel that their unease was understood; it would probably also have allowed them to concentrate on learning, rather than on controlling their emotions.

One of the most essential areas for education and training for both family and professionals is communication. However well a professional understands the family perspective in theory, if he or she cannot communicate that knowledge it is unlikely to make a difference in the relationship. Similarly, a family caregiver must be able to understand professional priorities, put his or her concerns into language that a professional will understand, and be able to ask questions, repeatedly if necessary, until the answer is understood.

Communication is not just talking back and forth; more important, it involves listening to another's spoken words and for another's unspoken fears or questions. Some essential aspects of communication can be taught, and today these skills are more likely to be incorporated into professional education. Yet most of the courses and workshops focus on physician-patient communication and not on communication with family caregivers. Although some elements are similar, some are different. Family caregivers may be superb communicators about the patient's care but never mention any of their own problems or concerns. These discussions require patience, sensitivity, compassion, and discretion.

They also require attention to the perhaps unspoken concerns of patients and families, which may not be the same as those of professionals. In a study of end-of-life care in Oregon all three interviewed groups—patients, families, and providers—ranked "clear decision making and preparation for death" as highly valuable (Steinhauser et al. 2000). Freedom from pain was ranked highest, and dying at home was least important. Of the three groups that participated in the survey, physicians were more often concerned about the biomedical aspects of care, while patients and families considered psychosocial and spiritual issues to be as important as physiological ones.

Palliative care teams deal with particularly emotion-laded circumstances, but the need for good communication skills extends throughout health care. There are several successful communication models to adapt and replicate. Maggie Hoffman and Donna Appell's chapter describes their work in Project DOCC (Delivery of Chronic Care), which builds family communication with resident pediatricians into all aspects of their training program. Parents are trained to talk to doctors in technical language about their child's disability but also to portray the child and family in human terms. Another significant program is "Enhancing Family Caregivers' Ability to Care," created by the National Family Caregiver Association (NFCA) with the assistance of the National Alliance for Caregiving. This program trains workshop leaders from around the country in communication skills, focusing on core communication strategies applied to health care settings. Role playing is a key part of the workshops, which also provide family caregivers with check lists, fact sheets, how-to-guides, and other supplements to reinforce the lessons learned in the workshop.*

Project DOCC also exemplifies another important aspect of education and training. Resident pediatricians make home visits to see how families with disabled children actually function in the community; the home parent is assisted by another trained parent to make sure that the visit goes well. In the geriatric field home visits have become more common; there is simply no substitute for seeing how a family lives and copes with illness within their own surroundings (Boal, Kornmeyer, and Toberg 2004; and Levine 2003). Except for home care nurses and aides, most health care providers today have never visited a patient's home; their understanding of how families function with caregiving responsibilities is based almost entirely on their experiences in hospitals or other facilities. This is a significant disadvantage for physicians, who are the only providers who can authorize home care but who have no experience with what it actually entails for the home care team and the family caregivers who implement the orders. If it is at all possible, every education program for professionals which deals with family caregiving should have a home visit component.

A complementary strategy includes guided visits to health care facilities for family caregivers. Caregivers attending workshops held through a United Hospital Fund–sponsored project at the Brooklyn Hospital Wartburg Lutheran Home for the Aged identified the Emergency Department (ED) as a site that they wanted to visit because so many had had distressing experiences bringing their family member to the ED. A tour led by the head of the ED gave caregivers a better understanding of what staff members look for in decisions to admit or treat, who the key personnel are, and how to get and give information about the patient (Levine 2003).

Ideally, incorporation of family caregiver issues should take place at all lev-

---

*More information is available on the NFCA Web site: www.nfca.org.

els of professional education and should be collaborative. In this context Mezey calls for a closer partnership between academic nursing and home care nursing. In its emphasis on technological skills and specialization the profession of nursing has adopted much of the culture of medicine, yet patients and family caregivers often look to nurses for support, training, and communication. This basic aspect of nursing should receive much more emphasis in training, especially in strengthening family caregiver skills, improving caregivers' attention to their own health, and supporting families through end-of-life passages.

Finally, formal educational activities should be complemented by informal teaching in which experienced professionals can, by example and by explicit discussion, demonstrate sensitive ways to talk to families, find resources for them, and include them in decision making about the patient's care, just as they are included in the patient's life.

Policy

As the chapter by Judith Feder and Carol Levine points out, there is as big a gap between the cultures of health care bureaucracies and family caregivers as there is between the cultures of health care professionals and family caregivers. At times it seems as though the culture of bureaucracies dominates even that of professionals. Surpin and Hanley describe the creation of a job category, home care aide, as a result of Medicare legislation that separated "skilled" needs from "unskilled" needs and the resulting welter of regulation which so confuses family caregivers.

Because public programs such as Medicare and Medicaid as well as private insurance consider only the designated beneficiary as eligible for services, implementing a family-centered approach calls for fundamental change. And, because the United States does not have a comprehensive long-term care policy, minor shifts in one part of the system do not carry through to other parts. Policy proposals to date have by necessity been piecemeal. They have also reflected policy makers' ambivalence toward family caregivers; they want to provide enough help to keep families on the job and not create new drains on public funds. They also continue to fear that formal home care services will drive out the unpaid family care, despite numerous studies that demonstrate that this is not the case (Penning 2002).

Considering all the barriers, it is remarkable that any progress on policy has been made at all. The most significant achievement to date was the enactment of the National Family Caregiver Support Program in 2000, which provides money to the states to distribute to Area Agencies on Aging within their jurisdiction to set up programs for family caregivers. The programs may include information about available services and assistance in gaining access to them; individual counseling, support groups, and caregiver training; respite care; and supplemental services on a limited basis to complement the care given by family members.

A one-year review of policies, perceptions, and practices in ten states reveals both the program's limited successes and the problems (Feinberg, Newman, and Van Steenberg 2002). The report found little consensus among the states about recognizing families as a central component of a long-term care system. Providing explicit support for family and friends of frail elders represents a paradigm shift for the aging network. In addition, respondents disagreed about whether or not family caregivers should be considered clients or consumers in the long-term care system and have access to their own support services. Some Medicaid officials reported that they would like to help family caregivers but were prevented from doing so by stringent rules. Agency officials considered the level of funding—$140 million in the first year—too low to meet the multifaceted needs of family caregivers. On the positive side this program is the first federal attempt to assist family caregivers and may offer models that can be expanded in the future.

Other legislative proposals have not fared even this well. Federal tax credits have been suggested at different times without success; they have been criticized by advocates for the poor, who do not pay taxes, as favoring the middle class and by long-term care advocates as an inadequate solution to the need for a comprehensive policy. A Lifespan Respite bill was introduced in 2002 by Sen. Hillary Clinton (D-NY) and a bipartisan group of sponsors, but it failed to reach the Senate floor. It was reintroduced in 2003. This effort is notable for the attempt to build a coalition including advocates for parents of disabled children and family caregivers of elderly people.

Although there has been limited success on the federal front, several states have introduced programs with their own funding. California, Pennsylvania, and New Jersey are notable examples. California has a system of eleven Caregiver Resource Centers serving caregivers of adults with cognitive impairments and other chronic conditions administered not by the state's aging department, as is usually the case, but by its mental health and social services department. There is considerable flexibility at the local level to meet caregivers' needs, which include the need for respite, family consultation, support groups, caregiver education and training, and assistance in finding formal care providers. Many of the state programs are means tested, and some agencies limit eligibility to caregivers who have a relative already receiving services.

Some of the most important policies that could help caregivers are those that directly recognize the caregiver's needs, but others that might be equally helpful to caregivers are aimed at helping the patient. Perhaps the most far-reaching policy changes that would help family caregivers would be making Medicare more flexible and more family centered. The National Academy of Social Insurance (NASI) in 2003 proposed restructuring Medicare to make it more applicable to chronic care in the twenty-first century. In addition to covering prescription drugs and preventive health services, its recommendations included relaxing "the requirement that to be covered for home care, beneficiaries must be homebound" and covering "durable medical equipment with the specific intent of maintaining or restoring function." Additional recommendations were to "provide for assistive devices that compensate for sensory or neurological deficits" and to "support rehabilitation as a tool to improve, maintain, or slow the decline of function." Although these are benefits for the individual, they have an indirect financial and quality-of-life benefit for family caregivers. Specifically in regard to families, the NASI report recommended providing families information and education about Medicare policies and choices of health plans and providers and adding an explicit patient-family education benefit. Providers should be adequately compensated for family consultation as well.

Although couched in regulatory language, these recommendations implicitly recognize the culture gap described in this volume. What is important to most family caregivers and their ill or disabled relatives is function, quality of life, and the ability to participate as much as possible in normal family activities. What Medicare and other policy standards, as well as much of professional culture, are interested in is curing the patient or achieving continuous improvement in measurable increments—the acute care model, not the chronic care reality that most family caregivers face. It will take a paradigm shift of monumental proportions to make these changes, but at least the need to consider a major restructuring is being articulated.

The one aspect of the health care system in which family participation and impact are explicitly recognized is hospice, and Blustein and Rothman specifically suggest it is a model that might be adapted for other types of care. While hospice's philosophy clearly includes the family, its impact is limited because patients come to it so late in the course of their illness. A quarter of hospice patients stay less than a week (General Accounting Office 2000). There are also many regulatory and attitudinal barriers around eligibility for and acceptance of hospice. Even though the six-month period of terminal illness required by Medicare can be recertified, hospices are reluctant to accept patients with uncertain prognoses. Physicians are reluctant to bring up the option, and families are often reluctant to accept what they see as abandonment and loss of hope. Even with the full range of hospice services, family caregivers whose relatives die at home are largely responsible for the direct care. The importance of hospice for our purposes is not the precise nature of the program but the coming together of the professional and family culture around an agreed-upon goal of care and a process for assisting families through this final phase. If this can be done at the end of life, why can it not be done at earlier stages of illness or disability?

Given the major, life-changing responsibilities many family caregivers take on, and the resourcefulness with which they carry on, it is striking that their requests for assistance are so modest. While bureaucrats may envision a throng of angry caregivers demanding full-time paid help and release from all their responsibilities, in the few instances in which family caregivers have been asked what they need, the answers are typically quite modest. They either refuse to consider that they might need anything, when it is their relative who needs so much, or they may offer a diffident suggestion such as "I could use a few hours off once in a while" or "I wish there were a support group nearby." One of the defining aspects of the culture of caregiving seems to be a deep reluctance to acknowledge one's own limitations and vulnerabilities in the face of another's more desperate need. One of the goals of research, education, and policy should be to recognize and build on the resilience and strengths of caregivers while offering them acceptable options for assistance.

Conclusion

By breaking out of outdated notions and perceptions and reconceptualizing the relationship between families and the health care system as one of a cultural divide, this volume will, we hope, open a discussion of better ways to create humane and compassionate environments for care. This is not just a matter of benevolence; it is also a matter of justice. As a recent report from the World Health Organization asserted, "A society that treats its most vulnerable members with compassion is a more just and caring society for all" (2002, 5).

REFERENCES

Boal, J., S. Korn-Meyer, and L. Toborg. (2004). "Mount Sinai's Geriatric Home Visiting Program." In Levine, C., ed., *Always On Call: When Illness Turns Families into Caregivers,* ed. C. Levine, 2d ed. Nashville: Vanderbilt University Press.

Feinberg, L. F., S. L. Newman, and C. Van Steenberg. (2002). *Family Caregiver Support: Policies, Perceptions and Practices in 10 States since Passage of the National Family Caregiver Support Program.* San Francisco: Family Caregiver Alliance.

Forster, A. J., H. J. Murff, J. F. Peterson, T. K. Gandhi, and D. W. Bates. (2003). "The Incidence and Severity of Adverse Events Affecting Patients after Discharge from the Hospital." *Annals of Internal Medicine* 138(3):161–67.

General Accounting Office. (2000). "Medicare: More Beneficiaries Use Hospice, yet Many Factors Contribute to Shorter Length of Stay." Washington, D.C.: General Accounting Office.

Levine, C., ed. (2004). *Family Caregivers on the Job: Moving beyond ADLs and IADLs.* New York: United Hospital Fund.

———. (2003). *Making Room for Family Caregivers: Seven Innovative Hospital Programs.* New York: United Hospital Fund.

Monahan, D.J., and K. Hopkins. (2002). "Nurses, Long-Term Care, and Eldercare: Impact on Work Performance." *Nursing Economics* 20(6):266–72.

National Academy of Social Insurance. (2003). *Medicare in the 21st Century: Building a Better Chronic Care System.* Washington, D.C.: National Academy of Social Insurance.

Penning, M. J. (2002). "Hydra Revisited: Substituting Formal for Self- and Informal In-Home Care among Older Adults with Disabilities." *Gerontologist* 42(1):4–16.

World Health Organization. (2002). *Ethical Choices in Long-Term Care: What Does Justice Require?* Geneva: World Health Organization.

Index